AF552495

UNDERSTANDING PHYSIOLOGY

UNDERSTANDING PHYSIOLOGY

By

Ashok Kumar
Dept. of Zoology
Bundelkhand University
Campus Department
Jhansi (India)

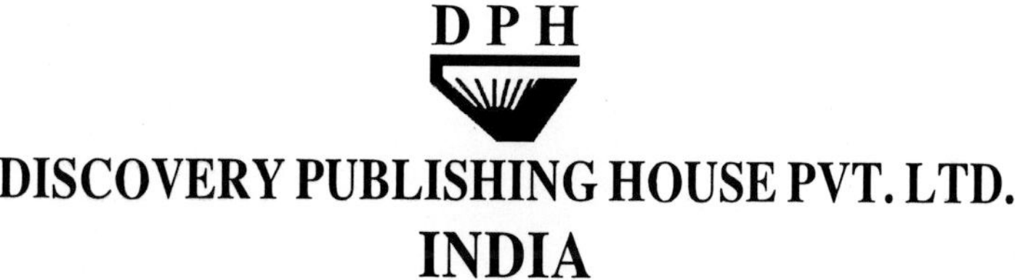

DISCOVERY PUBLISHING HOUSE PVT. LTD.
INDIA

Published by:

DISCOVERY PUBLISHING HOUSE PVT. LTD.
4383/4B, Ansari Road, Darya Ganj
New Delhi-110 002 (India)
Phone : +91-11-23279245; 23253475; 43596065
E-mail : discoverybooksindia@gmail.com
discoverypublishinghouse@gmail.com
namitwasan9@gmail.com
web : www.discoverypublishinggroup.com

***First Published:* 2009**
***Reprinted:* 2022**

ISBN: 978-81-8356-478-6

Understanding Physiology

Printed at:
Infinity Imaging Systems
Delhi

Preface

The present title "Understanding Physiology" has been written for those students interested in careers in diverse fields of biological sciences. It provides a structured approach to learning by covering all the important topics in a uniform, systematic format. The book has been comprehensively designed incorporating recent advances in this fast moving field. It also provides accessible information on physiology in compact form for undergraduate students in biology and related life sciences. It is intelligible to the educated layman, though it deals with some complex ideas. It is an adequate text for all the requirements of students in this area. In addition, busy lecturers who require a quick reference compendium will find it useful, particularly for tutional planning. Simple, yet hopefully clear figures and tables are provided throughout the book.

The over-riding goal of this book, and indeed of the whole *Understanding series*, is to present the essential information concerning physiology in a compact, readily accessible form which leads itself to student learning and revision. The convergence of various approaches has generated a rich panorama of detail, the significance of which we are still attempting to unraval. The present text has been written as an introduction to this rapidly growing field.

To make the work more comprehensive and informative, the author has consulted many authoritative books, research journals, abstracts, monographs etc., so there can be no claim to originality except in the manner of treatment.

The author expresses his thanks to his friends and colleagues whose continue inspirations have initiated him to bring out this book.

The author expresses his gratitude to Mr. Wasan and staff of M/s Discovery Publishing House Pvt. Ltd. for their whole hearted cooperation in the publication of this book.

In the mean time, the author will remain sincerely responsible for any shortcomings of the book and be grateful to the readers for their suggestions and constructive criticism for the continuous betterment of the book. He takes this opportunity to appeal to the readers to send their suggestions straightaway to his Publisher.

Author

Contents

1

INTRODUCTION

Even those of us who have most marveled at the exquisite architecture of an orchid flower, or who are as content as Leeuwenhoek to watch the intricate and varied movements of a *Paramecium* and its neighbors, approach the subject of the biology of our own systems with a quickened interest. Indeed for some, student and scientist alike, the principal and perhaps the only reason for studying "lower forms" is the extent to which such studies bear directly on human welfare. But as *Escherichia coli*, T2 and T4 bacteriophages, and *Drosophila* remind us, there is no way to study only the human species, any more than it is possible to study only a fruit fly.

In this section of the book, which deals with vertebrate physiology, we shall examine *Homo sapiens* as an example of an animal organism. This one species, however, will not command our full attention. First, we shall rely heavily on your understanding of the principles governing such matters as surface and volume, diffusion and osmosis, and gas exchange and water balance, which were discussed and exemplified in earlier chapters.

Second, in the chapters that follow, we shall introduce numerous examples from other organisms that illuminate our central theme-human physiology. Finally, we shall continue to emphasize broad principles rather than lose our way in a mass of details and intricate terminology. Because we are part of a continuum of nature, it is logical to study other animals in order to understand the human animal; it is equally logical to study the human animal (now one of the best understood) in order to gain a deeper understanding of animal life in general.

In 1966, George Gaylord Simpson, one of the leading modern students

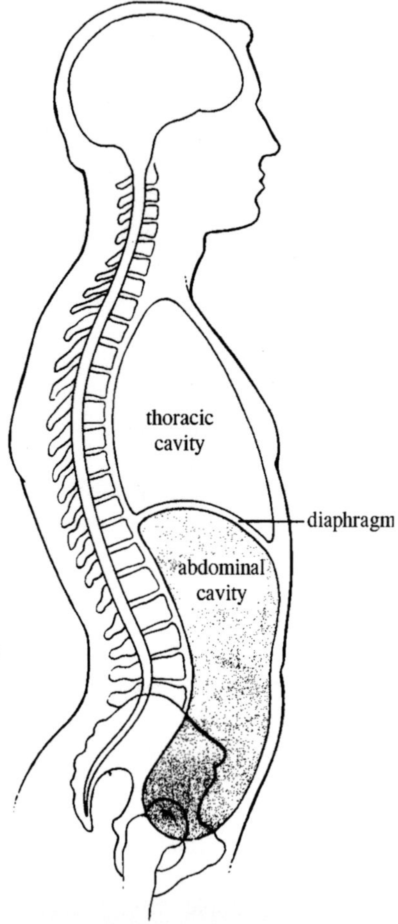

Figure 1.1: Humans, like other vertebrates, are characterised by a dorsal nervous system enclosed in vertebrae and the skull.

of evolution, wrote: The question "What is man?" is probably the most profound that can be asked by man. It has always been central to any system of philosophy or of theology. We know that it was being asked by the most learned humans 2,000 years ago, and it is just possible that it was being asked by the most brilliant australopithecines 2 million years ago. The point I want to make now is that all attempts to answer that question before 1859 are worthless and that we will be better off if we ignore them completely.

Some of us may not accept Simpsori s dismissal of pre-Darwinian philosophy, but there are few who would not agree about the relevance of his statement to human biology. The human being is a vertebrate, and as such has a bony, articulated (jointed) endoskeleton that supports the body and grows as it grows. The spinal cord, which is dorsal, is surrounded by bony segments, the vertebrae, and the brain is enclosed in a protective casing, the skull.

The skeleton is moved by means of muscles. As in other vertebrates, and most invertebrates as well, the human body contains a cavity, or coelom. In humans, the coelom is divided into two parts, the thoracic cavity and the abdominal cavity. These are separated by a dome-shaped muscle, the diaphragm. The thoracic cavity contains the heart, the lungs, and the upper portion of the digestive tract.

The abdominal cavity contains the stomach, intestines, liver, and other organs. Human beings are also mammals. One of the most important characteristics of mammals is that they are warm-blooded. More precisely, they are homeotherms; that is, they maintain a high and relatively constant body temperature. As a consequence, mammals (and birds, which are also homeotherms) are able to achieve and sustain levels of physical activity and mental alertness generally far greater than those of animals whose temperatures rise and fall with those of their external environment.

A concomitant of homeothermy is a high metabolic rate, which requires relatively large and constant supplies of food (fuel) molecules and oxygen. Mammals have other important characteristics. They have hair or fur rather than scales or feathers. All mammals (except the monotremes) give birth to live young, as distinct from laying eggs, which all birds and most fish, amphibians, and reptiles do. They nurse their offspring, which involves a relatively long period of parental care. This degree of parental care is correlated with a relatively long learning period (as contrasted, for example, with insects, most species of fish, and amphibians and reptiles, most of which are independent from the moment they hatch from the egg).

There is a tendency among the large mammals, in particular, toward fewer young per litter and an even longer period of parental care. Humans, for instance, rarely have more than two surviving young per birth, only two mammary glands with which to nurse them, and an extraordinarily long period of infancy and childhood, with dependency on parents often lasting well past physical maturity. As a consequence, at least in part, of homeothermy and the long learning period, mammals are, in general, by far the most intelligent of all groups of organisms.

They have the most highly developed systems for receiving, proces-

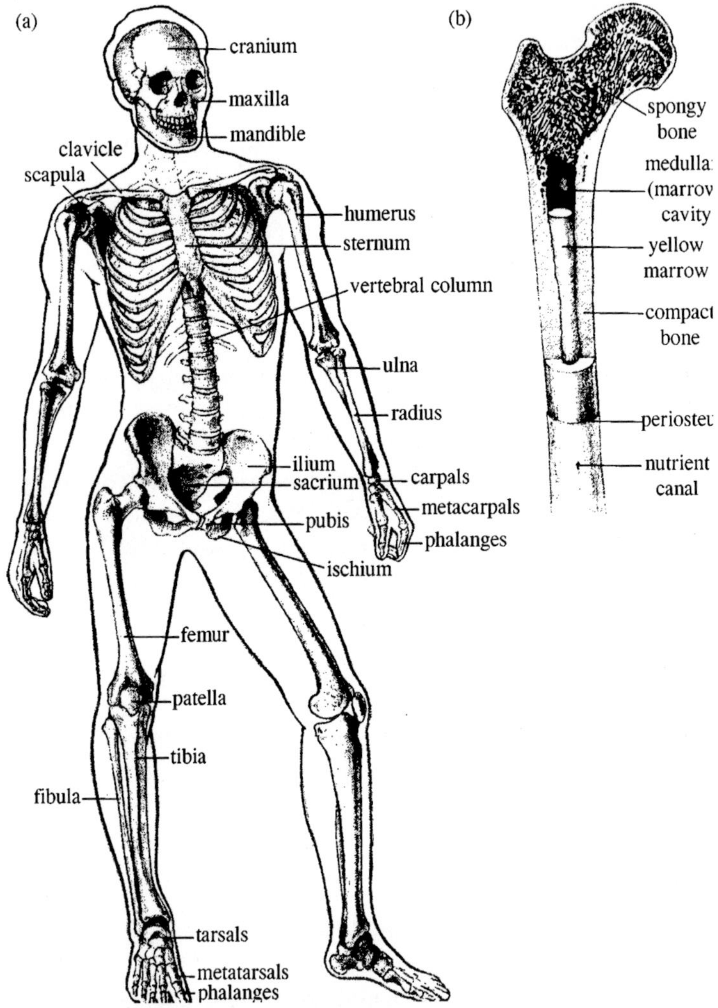

Figure 1.2: (a) The skeleton of a human adult contains 206 bones. Twenty nine are in the skull, including 14 face bones and six small bones (ossides) of teh ears. Ther are 27 bones in each hand and 26 in each foot. (b) The ends of long bones such as this femur consist of spongy none, in which there are large spaces, surrounded by compact bone.

sing, and correlating information from the environment (although, as we noted in other chapter of this book, in complexity and variety of sense organs, they are in some cases surpassed by some of the invertebrates). The class Mammalia comprises a large number of different species, ranging from whales and dolphins, bats, moles and hedgehogs, hippopotamuses, zebras and rhinoceroses, to gorillas and marmosets.

Among the members of this class, the human being is distinguished first by being versatile rather than specialised. A human cannot run as fast as a deer, swim as gracefully as a seal, or swing from branch to branch with the agility of a gibbon. But he or she can, if adequately motivated, run several kilometers, swim a river, and climb a tree-and few other mammals can do all three. Finally, for better or worse, *Homo sapiens* is by far the most intelligent of all mammalian species.

CELLS AND TISSUES

The human body, like that of all other complex animals, is made up of a great variety of different cells. Each of these cells is, to some extent, an independent entity. Each needs oxygen, glucose (or some other source of carbon and energy), amino acids, and small amounts of other substances (such as iron). Each needs to dispose of carbon dioxide and other wastes.

Human physiological processes, like those of any other organism, are concerned with providing second-by-second, 24-hour-a-day service to each of these billions of cells. Although they greatly resemble one-celled organisms in their requirements, the cells of an animal body differ from one-celled organisms in that they develop and function as part of an organised whole. As we shall see, cells are organised into *tissues*, groups of cells similar in structure and function.

Different kinds of tissues, united structurally and coordinated in their activities, form *organs*. The eye, with its many different types of fibers, is an example of an organ. Organs that function together in an integrated and organised way make up *organ systems*. The digestive system, for example, is composed of a number of different organs, each of which carries out a specific activity that contributes toward the overall process.

Because the focus of this section is on the various functions of the body, we shall be examining it principally in terms of organ systems. Although experts can distinguish more than 100 different types of cells in the human body, they customarily classify them in terms of only four tissue types: (1) epithelial, (2) connective, (3) muscle, and (4) nerve.

Epithelial Tissue

Epithelial tissue consists of a continuous sheet of cells that provides a protective covering of the whole body and contains various sensory nerve endings. It also forms the lining membranes of internal organs, cavities, and passageways. Hence, as a moment's reflection will reveal, everything that goes into and out of the body must pass through epithelial

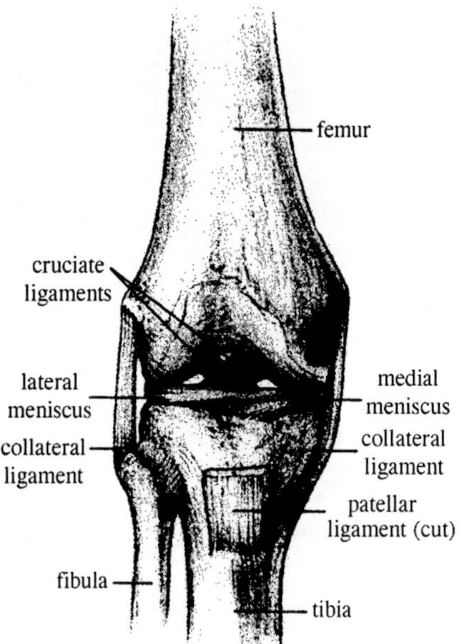

Figure 1.3: A knee is a hinge joint between the femur and the tibia, covering which is the "knee cap" or pratella.

cells. One surface of the epithelial sheet is always attached to an underlying layer, called the basement membrane, composed of a fibrous polysaccharide material produced by the epithelial cells themselves.

Epithelium is classified according to the shape of the individual cells as squamous, cuboidal, or columnar. It may consist of only a single layer of cells (simple epithelium), as found in the inner lining of the circulatory system, or several layers (stratified epithelium), as found in the epidermis of the skin.

The epithelium of the body cavities and passageways frequently contains modified epithelial cells that secrete mucus, which lubricates the surfaces. *Glands* are special types of epithelial tissue; gland cells produce specific substances, such as perspiration, saliva, hormones, or digestive enzymes. Glandular epithelium is composed of cuboidal or columnar epithelial cells.

Connective Tissue

Connective tissue binds together and supports the other three kinds of tissue. Unlike epithelial tissue cells, the cells of connective tissue are widely separated from one another by large amounts of intercellular substances. The intercellular substances include: (1) connecting and supporting fibers, such as collagen, which is a major component of skin,

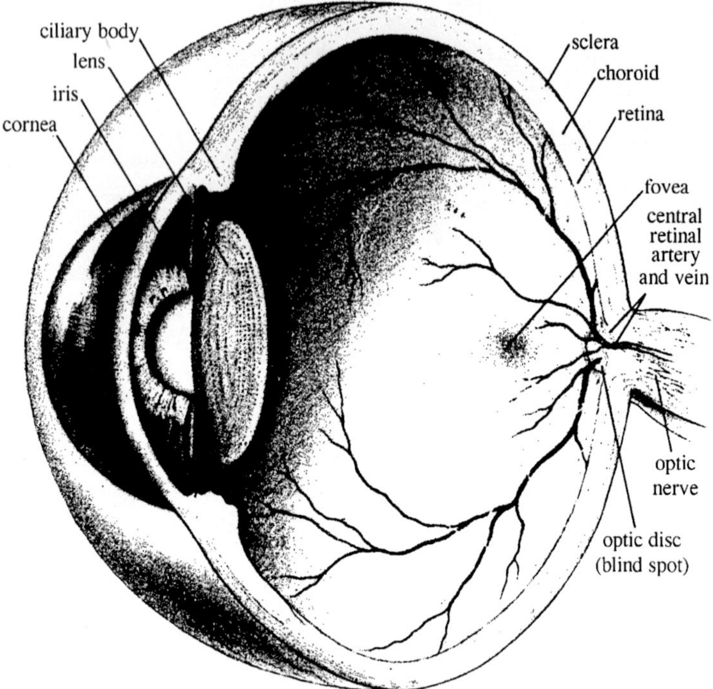

Figure 1.4: The eye is acomplex organ composed of three layers of tissue, which form a fluid-filled sphere.

tendons, ligaments, and bones; (2) elastic fibers, which are often found in the walls of hollow, distensible organs, such as the stomach and the uterus; and (3) reticular fibers, which form networks inside solid organs, such as the liver. All of these fibers are embedded in a matrix, or ground substance, that is more or less fluid and amorphous (without any shape or form).

Bone, like other connective tissues, consists of cells, fibers, and ground substance. It is unlike the others in that the collagen fibers are impregnated with hard crystals. Bone tissue is amazingly strong and light; our bones make up only about 18 percent of our weight.

Blood and lymph are connective tissues in which the matrix is plasma. The characteristic cells of blood and lymph are described in other chapter of this book.

Muscle Tissue

About 40 percent of our body's weight is made up of muscle tissue. There are two general types: smooth muscle and striated muscle, so

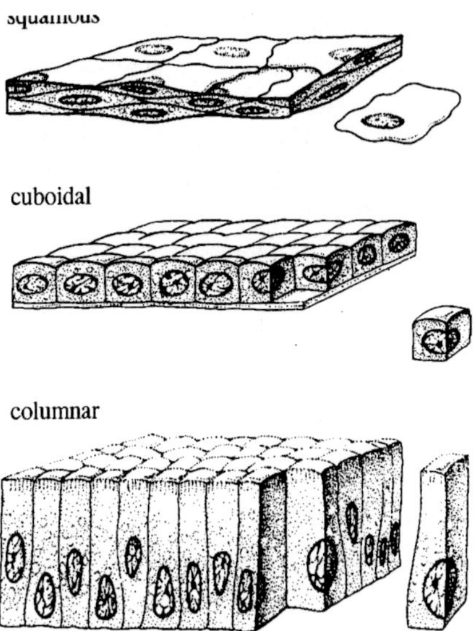

Figure 1.5: The three types of epithelial cells that cover the inner and outer surfaces of the body. Squamous cells, which usually perform a protective function, make up the outer layers of the skin and the lining of the mouth and other mucous membranes.

called because of its striped appearance. Striated muscle is the type of muscle that moves the skeleton; skeletal striated muscle is sometimes called voluntary muscle, since we can move it at will. Cardiac (heart) muscle is also striated muscle. Smooth muscle surrounds the walls of the internal organs, such as the digestive organs, uterus, and bladder; it is sometimes called involuntary muscle.

In this discussion, we shall focus on skeletal muscle because it is the subject of much current research, and much of what we know about the other forms of muscle is inferred from what has been learned about skeletal muscle. Also, studies of the machinery of skeletal muscle, involving as they do both electron microscopy and biochemistry, have brought scientists tantalizingly close to visualising the precise role of the individual molecules.

Muscle Action

Skeletal muscles, like all muscles, act by contracting. A skeletal muscle is typically attached to two or more bones, either directly or by means of the tough strands of connective tissue known as tendons. Some of these tendons, such as those that connect the finger bones and their muscles in the forearm, may be very long. When the muscle contracts, the bones move around a joint, which is held together by ligaments and contains a lubricating fluid. Most of the skeletal muscles of the body work in antagonistic pairs, one muscle flexing, or bending, the joint, and the other extending, or straightening, it.

A muscle, such as the biceps, consists of bundles of muscle fibers-often hundreds of thousands of fibers-held together by connective tissue. Each fiber is a single cell with many nuclei. These fibers are very large cells-50 to 100 micrometers in diameter and, often, several centimeters long. They are surrounded by an outer cell membrane that has been given the special name of sarcolemma.

Embedded in the cytoplasm of each muscle cell (fiber) are some 1,000 to 2,000 smaller structural units; they appear ribbonlike in electron micrographs but they are actually cylindrical strands. These strands, which are called *myofibrils* (from myo, the prefix for "muscle"), run parallel for the length of the cell. The nuclei are crowded to the periphery of the cytoplasm by the myofibrils and can typically be found at the cell surface, just beneath the sarcolemma.

Each myofibril is, in turn, composed of units called *sarcomeres*.

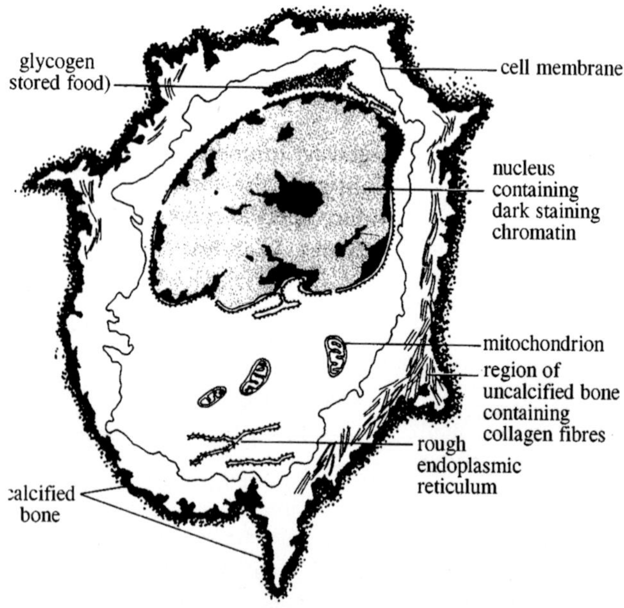

Figure 1.6: Electron micrograph and diagram of a bone cell (osteocyte). Young bone cells (osteoblasts) produce the intercellular bone matrix, an organic material consisting of collagen fibers and an unstructured ground substance. This matrix gradually calcifies and hardens.

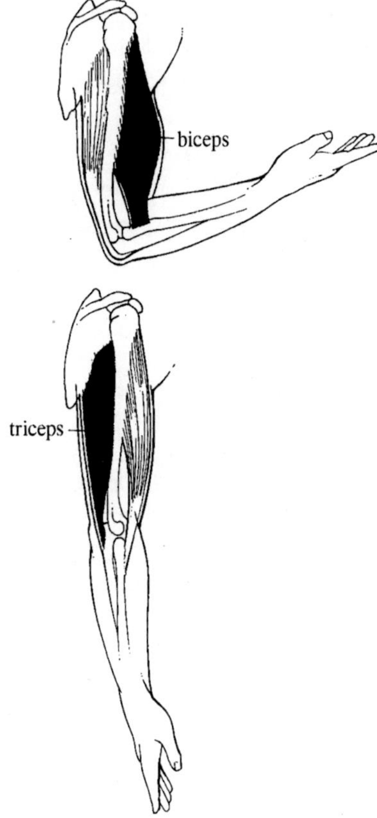

Figure 1.7: Muscles attached to bone move the vertebrate endoskeleton. They often work in an tagonistic pairs, with one relaxing as the other contracts.

The repetition of these units gives the muscle its characteristic striated pattern.

Figure elsewhere in this chapter shows a sarcomere as seen in a longitudinal section of muscle. Each sarcomere is about 2 or 3 micrometers in length. The Z line is the dense black line seen in the electron micrograph; the I band is the relatively clear, broad stripe that the Z line bisects; and the A band is the large, dense stripe in the center of the sarcomere bisected by the central H zone. As the diagram shows, each sarcomere is composed of two types of filaments running parallel to one another. The thicker filaments in the central portion of the sarcomere are composed of a protein known as myosin; the thinner-filaments are made of actin, also a protein. The Z line is where the actin filaments from adjacent sarcomeres interweave.

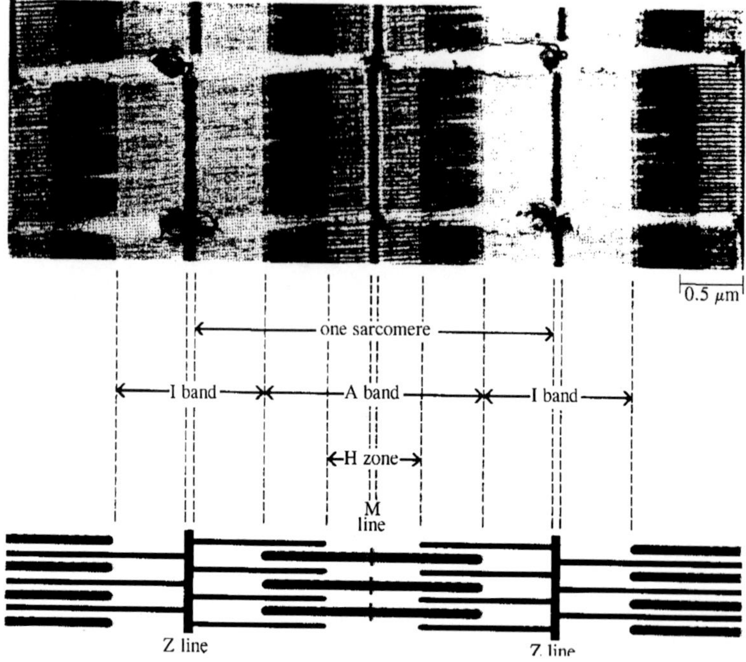

Figure 1.8: Electron micrograph and diagram of a sarcomere, the contractile unit of muscle. Eachsarcomere is composed of an array of thick and thin protein filaments arranged longitudinally.

Muscles function by contracting. From the cell physiologist's point of view, the exciting feature of the sarcomere is that it is the contractile machine. When muscle is stimulated, the thin (actin) filaments of the sarcomere slide past the thick (myosin) filaments. Since the thin filaments are anchored into each Z line, this causes each sarcomere to shorten, and thus the myofibril as a whole contracts. According to the current hypothesis, cross bridges between the thick and thin filaments form, break, and re-form rapidly, as one filament "walks" along the other.

Actin and Myosin

The actin strands in muscle are composed, it has been found, of many smaller globular subunits assembled in a long chain. As shown in Figure elsewhere in this chapter, each thin filament is composed primarily of two such actin chains wound around each other.

The myosin molecule has the longest protein chains known, each one consisting of some 1,800 amino acid units. Each long protein chain has a globular structure at one end. The myosin molecule consists of two of these chains wound around each other, with the globular "heads"

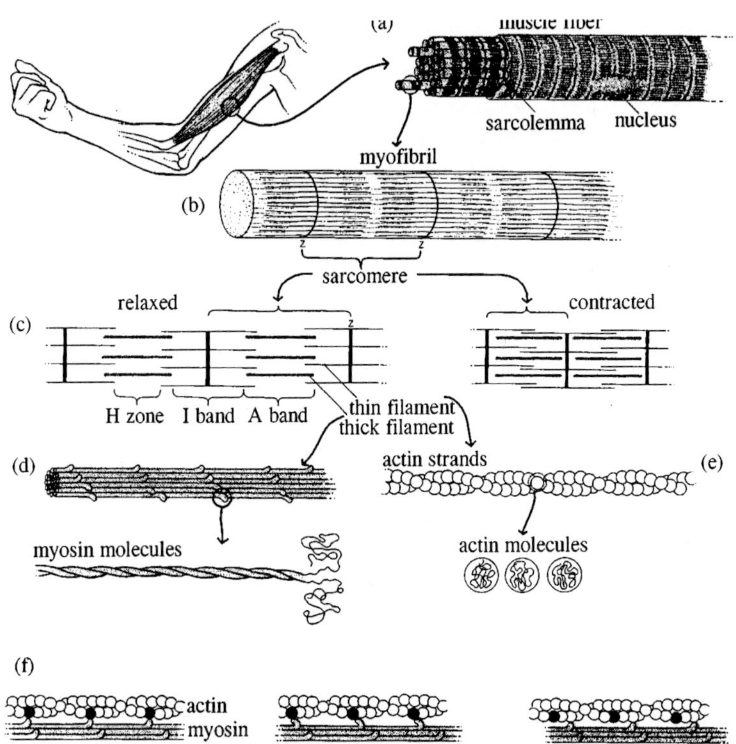

Figure 1.9: Skeletal muscle is composed of individual muscle cells, the muscle fibers. These are cylindrical cells, often many centrimeters long, with numerous nuclei.

free. The thick filaments, in turn, are composed of bundles of myosin molecules. These globular heads have two crucial functions: They are the binding sites that link the actin and myosin molecules, and they also act as enzymes to split ATP to ADP, thus providing the energy for muscle contraction.

To sum up, when a muscle fiber is stimulated, the thin (actin) filaments slide between the thick (myosin) filaments, and ATP is hydrolysed to ADP in the process. The sarcomeres shorten and the fibers contract. If enough fibers contract, a whole muscle contracts, and the organism or part of the organism moves. Thus the intricate machinery of the sarcomere is, in essence, a mechanism for the conversion of chemical energy into kinetic energy, the energy of motion.

Smooth Muscle

Smooth muscle contracts much less rapidly than striated muscle, and its contractions are more prolonged. Smooth muscle is responsible for the movement of food along the intestinal tract, for example, and the emptying of the bladder and the constriction of small blood vessels to regulate blood flow.

Unlike striated muscle, smooth muscle consists of cells with single nuclei. These cells contain numerous fibrils that run lengthwise through the cell but are not arranged in any discernible pattern. Thus no striations are apparent. Like striated muscle, smooth muscle cells contain large amounts of actin and myosin, which are presumed, but not proved, to

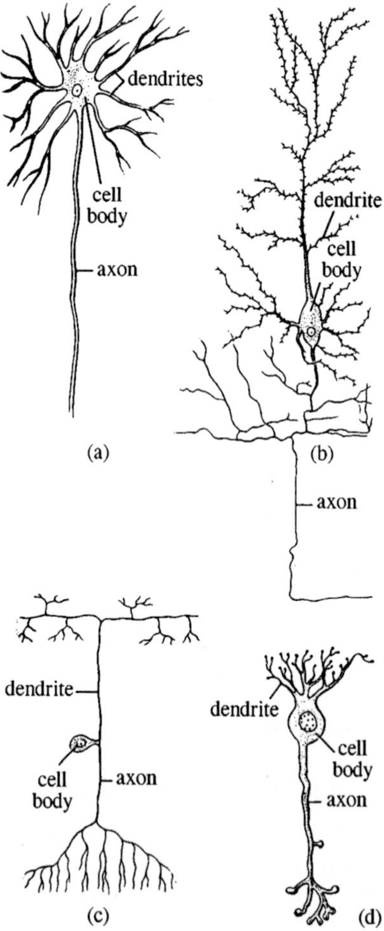

Figure 1.10: Four examples of neurons. Dendrites, which are characeristically multiple, transmit signals toward the neuron cell body, whereas axons, of which there is obnly one per cell, trasmit signals away fromt eh cell body of the neuron.

be in the fibrils and to play a role in the contraction of smooth muscle. Smooth muscle also requires ATP for contraction.

Nerve Tissue

The fourth major tissue type is nerve tissue. The basic units of nerve tissue are the neurons, or nerve cells, which make up about 10 percent of nerve tissue cells. Nerve cells receive and transmit signals from either the external or the internal environment. They also process this information and are responsible for the complex functions of consciousness, memory, and thought.

The other 90 percent of nerve tissue cells are glial cells, which support the neurons physically and also nourish, protect, and insulate them. (In terms of the bulk of nerve tissue, each cell type contributes about half.) A typical neuron consists of a cell body, which contains the nucleus and most of the metabolic machinery of the cell, and one or more long extensions, or processes (axons and dendrites). Along these neuron processes, nerve impulses are transmitted from one part of the organism to another.

These cells are the most morphologically spectacular of the body's cells. Neurons may reach astonishing lengths. For example, the axon of a single motor neuron-a nerve cell that activates muscle-may extend from the spinal cord down the whole length of the leg to the toe. Or a sensory neuron-one that transmits sensations to the brainbased near the spinal cord may send a dendrite down to the toe and an axon up the entire length of the spinal cord to terminate in the lower part of the brain. In an adult human, such a cell might be close to 2 meters long (5 meters in a giraffe).

The cell bodies of neurons are often found in clusters. Clusters of neuron cell bodies within the brain and spinal cord are called *nuclei*; clusters of neuron cell bodies outside the brain and spinal cord are called *ganglia* (singular, ganglion).

Nerve bundles are composed of many nerve fibers from many neurons-usually hundreds and sometimes thousands. Each fiber is capable of transmitting separate messages, like the wires in a telephone cable.

ORGANS AND ORGAN SYSTEMS

Organs are composed of functionally related groups of tissue. The stomach, for example, is made up of layers of glandular epithelium (the stomach lining), connective tissue, nerves, blood vessels, and smooth muscle. Organ systems, in turn, generally comprise a number of organs that work together to accomplish a function necessary to maintain or continue the life of the organism. The stomach, for instance, is part of the digestive system. One of the major organ systems, the urinary system, is shown in Figure elsewhere in this chapter.

INTEGRATION AND CONTROL

The adult human body is composed of several hundred trillion cells of more than 100 kinds, grouped together in many different structural and functional units.

Moreover, each cell is also working for itself, breaking down glucose, making ATP, building and maintaining membranes and organelles, producing enzymes and other protein molecules, dividing or not dividing. Yet in order for the organism as a whole to survive, all of these cells, tissues, and organs have to function as a whole.

For example, do you recall what it feels like to be in an absolute rage? The physical characteristics of a rage result from a simultaneous discharge of many nerve fibers. Certain of these cause the blood vessels in the skin and intestinal tract to contract; this contraction increases the return of the blood to the heart, raising the blood pressure and sending more blood to the muscles.

The heart beats both faster and stronger, and the respiratory rate increases. The pupils dilate. The muscles underlying the hair follicles in the skin contract; this is probably a legacy from our furry forebears, which looked larger and more ferocious with their hair standing on end. The rhythmic movement of the intestine stops, and sphincters, the muscles at the end of the intestines and the opening of the bladder, relax; these reactions inhibit digestive operations, but the relaxing of the sphincters may also have the disconcerting consequence of causing involuntary defecation or urination.

Hormones are produced that cause the release of large quantities of sugar from the liver into the bloodstream; this sugar provides an extra energy source for the muscles. The adrenal glands pour out epinephrine (adrenaline). As a consequence, the body as a whole is prepared for "fight or flight"-or, at least, action that would have been appropriate at some stage in our cultural evolution.

However, response to the external environment is only a small part of the organisms need for integration of its many individual functional units. Equally complex and vital, although less obvious, activities are required for the constant regulation of the internal environment. This maintenance of a relatively constant internal environment is known as *homeostasis. As* we noted in Chapter 1, homeostasis-"staying the same"-is one of the chief characteristics of living organisms. It is by regulating the internal environment that organisms have been able to free themselves

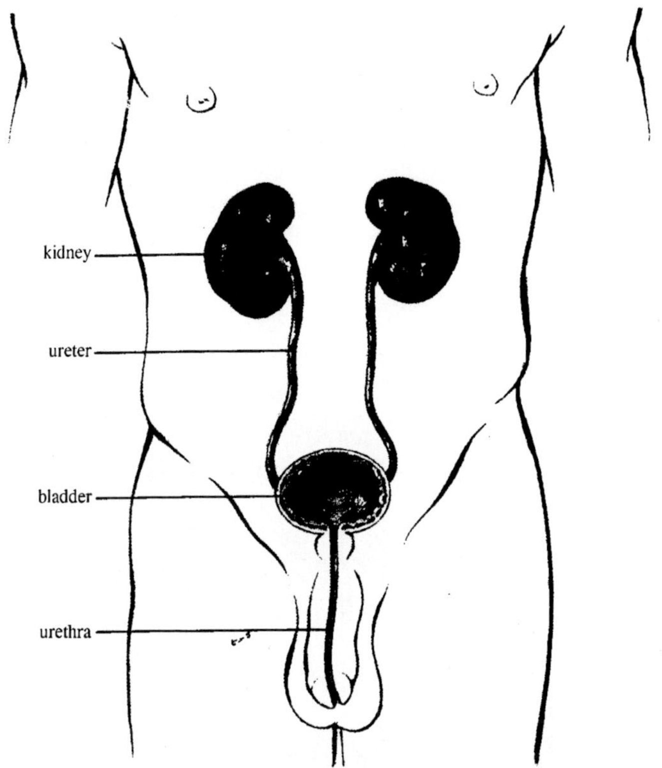

Figure 1.11: The urinary system is one of the major organ systems of the body. Fluids are processed in the kidneys, and waste products and water-the urine-pass along a pair of tubes, the ureters, to the bladder, where they are stored. Urine leaves the body by way of the urethra, which, in the male mammal, also serves as the passageway for semen.

to an increasing degree from the external environment, moving from salt water to fresh water, and from the water to the land and air.

Homeostasis is characteristic even of single cells and very simple organisms. In an organism as complex as *Homo sapiens,* it involves constant monitoring and regulation of a large number of different factors, such as oxygen and carbon dioxide, glucose and other nutrients, hormones, ions, pH, and temperature. Despite changes in the external environment and the organism's response to it, the concentrations of these substances in the body fluids remain relatively unchanged.

Virtually every cell, tissue, and organ in the body contributes in some way to this remarkable stability. The liver acts as a metabolic factory, removing organic molecules or adding them as they are needed. Oxygen for *ATP* production may be used rapidly, as during muscle exertion, or slowly, as during sleep, but the rates at which the lungs take in oxygen and the heart pumps blood are regulated so that the supply in the bloodstream available to the individual cells remains constant.

The kidney processes and removes just the right amount of wastes, water, and saltsand so on, down the long list of organs, tissues, and cells. Therefore, although we shall examine the various organ systems of the body one by one-as it is conventional to do-it is important to remember that all are acting in concert and that the function of each is affected by all the others.

2

INTERNAL ENVIRONMENT

About 200 years ago, Dr. Charles Blagden, then secretary of the Royal Society of London, proved that he was one of the most persuasive people on earth. He talked some friends into joining him, a small dog, and a steak in a room in which the temperature had been raised to 126°C (260°F). In fact, he managed to persuade his friends to stay in there for 45 minutes. (The dog and the steak had no choice.) At the end of this time, the men and the dog emerged unharmed, but the steak was cooked!

In addition to demonstrating his polemic powers, Blagden also showed that the bodies of animals are able to compensate for extreme physiological conditions and, in particular, that some living things can control their internal temperatures in the face of extreme external conditions. Since this early experiment, it has been found that animals can regulate a host of other internal physical and chemical states. The ability to hold things within certain limits should not be unexpected since the delicate processes of life would not be possible under wildly fluctuating conditions.

HOMEOSTASIS AND THE DELICATE BALANCE OF LIFE

Homeostasis is the tendency of living things to maintain a stable internal environment (from the Greek homios, same, and stasis, standing). The term is a bit misleading, however, because no living thing strictly maintains a constant internal environment. One reason is that maintaining such rigid constancy would place a great demand on the organism's metabolic machinery. Another reason is that some change must occur in order for things to stay the same. That is, as the environment changes, the body's internal processes must also shift in order to counteract the outside changes and keep the internal conditions stable. So cells do change as they constantly monitor, metabolise, and adapt. The result is a "steady state"-keeping the internal environment within certain limits-and that is what homeostasis is all about.

FEEDBACK SYSTEMS

Generally, the steady state is maintained by *feedback* mechanisms. Feedback occurs when the product of an action influences that action. Biologically, the most important kind of feedback action is called *negative feedback*. Negative feedback occurs when an increase in a system's product causes a slowdown of that system, or when a reduction of the product stimulates the system. One kind of "*cruise control*" on an automobile engine (a device that keeps the car moving at a certain speed) works because as the motor runs faster, valves are closed, causing the car to slow down.

As the car slows, the valves are reopened, and the car accelerates, keeping its speed within certain limits. Also, because of negative feedback mechanisms, you don't have to constantly nibble and fast to keep your blood sugars at the proper level. When blood sugars are low, the liver simply breaks down some of its stores of glycogen and releases glucose into the blood. As blood sugars rise, the liver is inhibited from breaking down glycogen, and instead converts the sugar to glycogen for storage.

Positive feedback works on the opposite principle: the product of a system increases the activity of that system. Using the example of an automobile, with positive feedback, accelerating the motor would tend to open the carburetor and cause the engine to run even faster. Such an engine might be revved to such limits that it would explode. Obviously, then, homeostasis operates primarily through the more delicate mechanisms of negative feedback, but this is not to say that living things are not sometimes subjected to positive feedback.

Positive feedback mechanisms in humans are sometimes associated with severe health problems. For example, if a person's temperature begins to rise above the normal 37°C, the body will activate corrective devices such as sweating and the opening of peripheral blood vessels (producing a heat-dissipating "*flush*"). However, at some point (usually at about 42°C), the negative feedback system breaks down, and a positive feedback begins. The high temperature begins to cause an increase in metabolic activity, which raises the heat, which increases metabolic activity, which can kill the unfortunate soul. (Positive feedback is the basis of the famed "*vicious circle.*") To better understand the principles of the two forms of feedback control, consider the operation of two simple storage tanks.

TEMPERATURE REGULATION

Many of the processes of life can occur only within a narrow range of temperatures, and the mechanisms by which this stabilization occurs may serve as a good example of homeostasis. First, we should note that an increase in temperature of only a few degrees can cause great leaps in the rate of chemical reactions. In nonliving material, the rule of thumb is: the rate of chemical reactions doubles for every 10°C increase in temperature. However, in living cytoplasm, such rules may not apply, and a change in temperature may have less effect.

Why is temperature so important to living things? Because of the severe effects of temperature extremes. At about - 1° to - 2°C, the water in cells freezes, causing ice crystals to form that may rupture delicate membranes. Also, with water tied up as ice, the remaining cell constituents may become so concentrated that they are unable to function properly. The result of such disruptions may be death.

At the other extreme, the upper temperature limit that life can withstand is apparently largely set by the temperature at which the hydrogen bonds holding proteins in their tertiary structures begin to break, thus unwinding (or denaturing) the protein. Because of the effects of temperature, most animals live in places that are not much colder than freezing or warmer than about 40°C. (Exceptions to such rules include certain algae, fungi, and bacteria that are able to live in hot springs at temperatures up to 80°C, and some species that cannot survive if "chilled" to the boiling point of water.)

Ectotherms

The *ectotherms*, or the so-called cold-blooded animals, include virtually all the vertebrates except birds and mammals (*ecto*, outside; *therm*, temperature). The ectotherms, therefore, include fish, amphibians and reptiles. Ectotherms do not physiologically regulate their body temperatures to any great extent.

Although they do produce metabolic heat, they have no efficient means of conserving it or of increasing or decreasing its production. If it is necessary to change their body temperatures, they may do so behaviourally simply by moving to a cooler or warmer place. In general, the saltwater fish have no great problems because the oceans rarely change in temperature more than a few degrees. However, freshwater fish living in the shallows are much more at the mercy of the elements. Furthermore, their efforts to thermoregulate behaviourally can put them at risk.

As they move from place to place, they may find themselves in danger of becoming landlocked. This means they risk overheating or drying out if they are unable to return to deeper water. Of course, freshwater fish that remain in deeper water suffer no such threat, but because of the low temperature at these depths, their metabolic rate is slow and so must be the pace of their lives.

Among land dwellers it's a different story. They face unbuffered temperatures and dry air with its rapidly changing temperatures. Somewhat surprisingly, amphibians have been able to adapt to such arid environs. One way they adjust is by simply moving overland to places with more agreeable temperatures. Some species may also bury themselves and thereby escape the drying air.

Other species that are exposed to extreme heat and drought have the ability to *estivate*—that is, to enter a form of summer "stupor" until reactivated by cool temperature and moisture. Toads in certain arid parts of Australia, in fact, have been known to remain buried for as long as two years while waiting for a good rain. The estivating toads have low metabolic rates, just as do hibernating animals, and therefore their food and oxygen requirements are low.

Land reptiles strongly rely on behavioural regulation, as do amphibians, they simply move to areas that are more appropriate to their needs. As with many other ectotherms, they also allow their body temperatures to drop with the cool of night. This results in a certain sluggishness in the morning because their metabolic rates have slowed accordingly.

If they are going to catch any food, however, they've got to warm up, and they quickly do so by utilising the warmth of the sun. Basking ectotherms are able to absorb the heat of the sun even when the air temperature is near freezing. As the day wears on, the animals may seek shade or turn to face the sun, which reduces the surface area exposed to its rays. During the hottest part of the day, some species may retreat underground, reappearing only in the cooler afternoon.

Endotherms

Birds and mammals comprise the *endotherms* (*endo*, inside), the so-called warm-blooded creatures. They have evolved physiological methods of keeping their body temperatures within very narrow limits. Their bodies can carry out biochemical activities more efficiently by having specialised to within a range of temperatures that is conducive to biochemical reactions.

Interestingly, both birds and mammals are descended from the reptiles. Mammals appeared at about the time the dinosaurs made their entrance, about 150 million years ago (the birds evolved a little later). While the great dinosaurs were thundering around the earth terrorizing everything in sight, the mammals were existing as tiny mouselike forms that probably terrorised only insects.

After the disappearance of the dinosaurs, the numbers of birds and mammals *burgeoned*. As they radiated out over the earth, invading newlyvacated niches, the endotherms began to change and specialise in innumerable ways. Nonetheless, both birds and mammals, having sprung from the same distant stock, had certain critical traits in common-traits related to temperature control.

First, they were well-insulated creatures, with their fur and feathers. Second, they had a more efficient four-chambered heart. Theirs was a powerful organ able to pump enough fuel and oxygen throughout the body to stoke the cells' metabolic furnaces. Remember, the cost of struggling against the environment to maintain a constant internal temperature would have been metabolically expensive and would have required increasingly efficient physiological mechanisms.

Since in endotherms, metabolic heat (a by-product of certain chemical reactions) travels from the inside out, bodies tend to be warmer toward the inside. Thus, if you should touch something that is 37° C (your body's internal temperature), it will feel warm because your skin is cooler than that. So, there is some variation from place to place in your body, and there is even some variation from time to time. (Your temperature usually falls a bit in the wee hours of the morning and rises in the early afternoon.) Because of the greater constancy in the deeper tissues, if you measure someone's temperature with a rectal thermometer, you will get not only his undivided attention, but a more precise reading as well.

Here I should add that there is some recent evidence suggesting that for those who are ill, aspirin or other fever-reducers may do more harm than good. It has been suggested that a slight rise in the body's temperature can render it inhospitable to temperature-sensitive viruses and bacteria. Physical exercise can also raise the body's temperature

Table 2.1 : Mammalian Responses to Temperature Stress

Stimulus	*Response*	*Effect*
Hot temperature	Sweating or panting	Evaporative heat loss
	Dilation of peripheral blood vessels	Heat lost from warm blood at body surface
	Changes in behaviour reduce heat generated	Increase heat loss or
Cold temperature	Constriction of peripheral blood	Reduce heat loss at body surface vessels
	Increased muscle activity (shivering)	increase heat production
	Secretion of thyroxine from thyroid gland and epinephrine from adrenal cortex increases metabolic rate	Increase heat production
	Changes in behaviour	Alter heat loss or heat production

and, some say, thereby stave off certain illnesses by rendering the body unsuitable for habitation by pathogens.

How does your body "know" its own temperature? The temperature is monitored by a delicate thermostat in the *hypothalamus* (an ancient part of the brain). Certain receptor cells monitor the temperature of the blood reaching the brain. If the blood is too warm, the hypothalamus initiates a chain of events that brings down the temperature. This is done in different ways in different animals, and both physiological and behavioural responses may be involved.

As body temperatures rise, humans and most other large animals sweat, and the evaporation cools them. Dogs pant and rapidly move cooling air over their large tongues and through their lungs. (They may also lie down under a tree-a behavioural response.) Cats are stimulated to lick themselves and are cooled by the evaporation of the saliva.

In some animals, including humans, peripheral blood vessels dilate, bringing warm blood to the surface of the skin where heat can be exchanged.

As the blood cools, the surface vessels contract, reducing heat loss over the skin's surface. The hypothalamus then signals the pituitary to direct the thyroid glands, located in the throat area, to release a hormone (called thyroxine) that increases metabolic rate. In addition, if the temperature of the blood in the brain should drop to dangerous temperatures, the hypothalamus will direct the adrenal glands to secrete epinephrine (adrenalin), thereby increasing the metabolic rate and raising the body's temperature.

If the temperature continues to drop, shivering begins, causing the surface muscles to work and to increase their metabolism, thereby producing more heat and using more energy. Have you noticed that you eat more in the winter? Why do you suppose that is?

Occasionally the body's thermostat is "turned up," and fever results. No one really knows how fever occurs, but infection seems to trigger the release of *pyrogens* ("*heat causers*") that elevate the body's temperature. Before fever, when the temperature is still normal, the body begins to behave as if it were cold. (The *hypothalamus* responds as if it were detecting cold.)

Blood vessels in the skin contract ("You look pale; do you feel well?"), and shivering may begin as the rate of metabolism increases. All these things can act together to bring on higher temperatures. Finally, the temperature temporarily stabilizes at its new, higher setting. When the fever breaks, the opposite responses occur. The skin becomes flushed and sweating occurs until enough heat is lost to restore the body to normal temperature.

Just as your body's temperature is kept within narrow limits, so are other physiological factors. In fact, every activity involving growth and maintenance is controlled by complex regulatory mechanisms. One of the clearest examples of such control involves water balance. You have probably heard that the body to which you are attached is composed mostly of water, and physiologists have glibly quoted rather precise numbers to tell you just what the percentage is. How can they be so sure? Do they include the bodies that have just completed marathons, or those that have been drunk for three days? Not normally, but still they are confident because they are aware of the delicate and intolerant mechanisms of the kidneys.

THE EXCRETORY SYSTEM

The Nitrogenous Wastes

All animals have the problem of getting rid of metabolic wastes, or "cell garbage." Much of this waste is in the form of excess nitrogens that are left over when proteinaceous foods are *metabolised* in this process, the proteins are stripped of their nitrogens and the remainder of the molecules are converted into whatever is needed, such as glucose. This leaves the nitrogens to combine with other elements, forming poisonous nitrogenous by-products.

The nitrogen atoms that are stripped from the proteins are not utilised in either the anaerobic or aerobic energy cycles. Once free, they usually pick up three hydrogens-and NH_3 is *ammonia*, a deadly poison. The problem, then, is how to dispose of the ammonia. However, ammonia is so poisonous that it must be highly diluted in order to be handled by the body, and in water-conserving species, any such dilution would result in the loss of too much water.

The problem is solved by the addition of components of carbon dioxide to the ammonia, forming *urea*, a less toxic molecule that the body can handle in higher concentrations. A moderately dilute urea is then passed out of the body as *urine*.

Many terrestrial species, notably the egg-laying birds and the insects, have a particular need to conserve water, so they have developed the means to convert ammonia to an insoluble nitrogenous product called *uric acid*. The uric acid is excreted almost as a dry paste in some species. The major waste products of metabolism in fish (ammonia), birds (uric acid), and mammals (urea)* are:

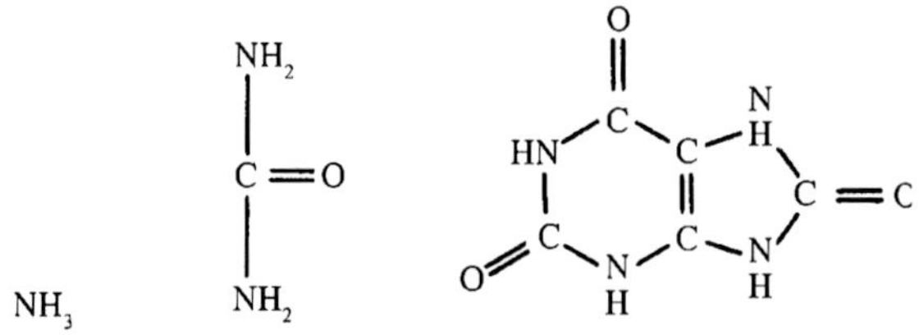

NH_3 — ammonia

NH_2–C(=O)–NH_2 — urea

uric acid

SOLUTIONS TO THE WATER PROBLEM

One of the great problems in the development of excretory systems was how to flush metabolic wastes from the body without losing too much water. The evolutionary solutions, we shall see, have been quite diverse.

Vertebrates have evolved a number of ways of ridding the body of metabolic wastes and maintaining proper internal water levels. For example, freshwater fish, like freshwater protozoa, live in a *hypotonic*

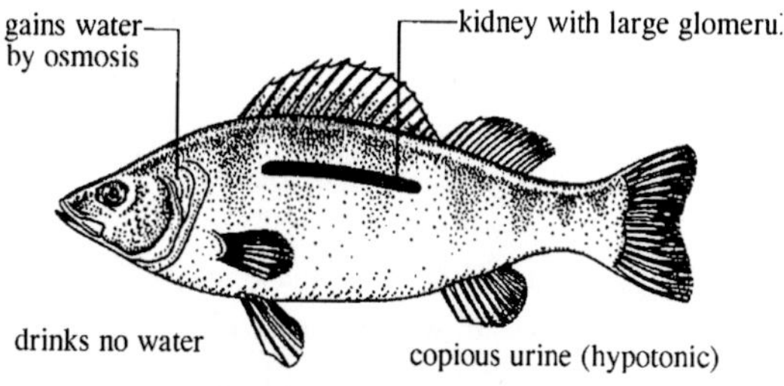

FRESH-WATER FISH

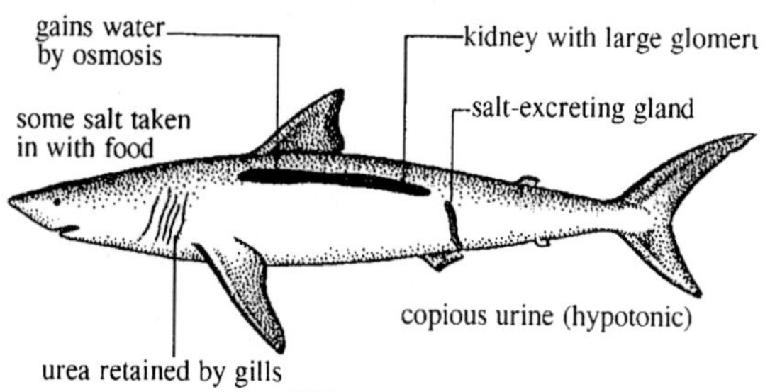

SHARK

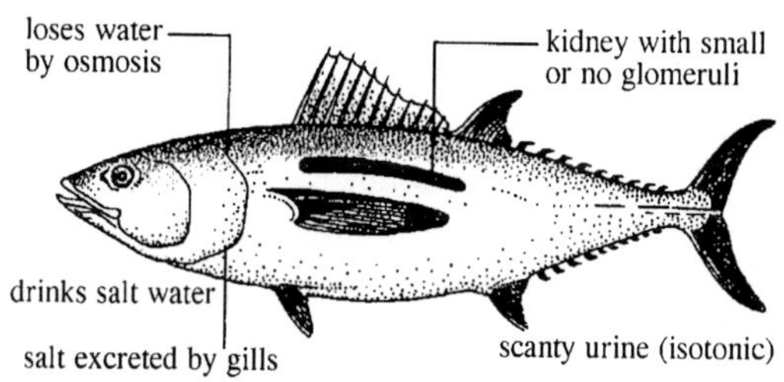

SALT-WATER BONY FISH

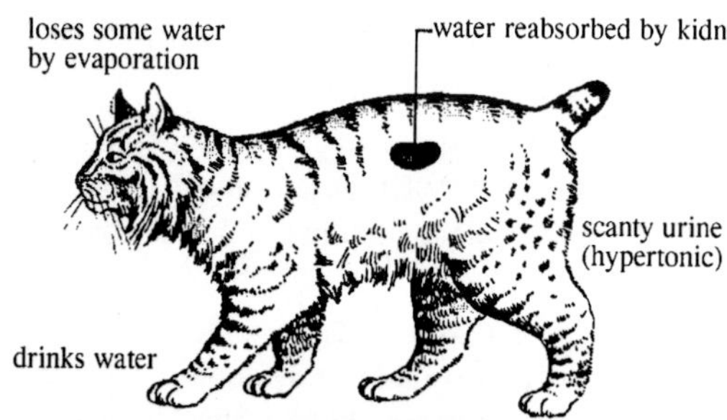

TERRESTRIAL ANIMAL

Figure 2.1 : Regulation of water and salt balances in a representative group of animals. Water enters the freshwater fish by osmosis. Great amounts of fluid cross its glomeruli daily, and it excretes large amounts of water in its urine.

medium; that is, the concentration of particles in their body fluids is higher than that in the surrounding water. Hence, water tends to move into their bodies by osmosis. One means by which they rid themselves of excess water is through a great number of tiny blood vessels in their kidneys.

These blood vessels are coiled into tiny clumps that keep the blood in one area for an extended time and are called *glomeruli* (singular, *glomerulus*). We'll consider the structure of the glomeruli shortly, but suffice it to say here that, in general, they provide a large surface area through which fluids leave the blood to be collected in the kidney.

The metabolic waste in freshwater fish is also highly dilute. This is to be expected since they have no problem finding enough water to flush out their wastes. Saltwater animals, interestingly enough, have the same problem as desert animals: conserving water. Seawater is a hypertonic medium; that is, its concentration of solutes is higher than the fluids in the marine animal's body.

Hence, these animals tend to lose water by osmosis. As a result, many have developed smaller glomeruli, so that there is less opportunity for water to filter out as it passes through the kidney. Saltwater fish replace the lost water by drinking seawater. They rid themselves of the excess salts from seawater by excreting some across the gills and some in the urine. Other salts are never absorbed and pass out in the feces. In other animals, specialised gills or other structures may also eliminate nitrogenous waste as blood passes through them.

Most sharks and rays in the ocean have a different strategy: they retain some urea, or waste, in their blood. This raises the osmotic pressure of their body fluid so that it is closer to that of seawater. Thus they sidestep many problems of the excretion of both water and metabolic wastes. (Various solutions to different water and nitrogen problems.)

Selected Invertebrate Excretory Systems

Different species may dispose of nitrogenous metabolic wastes in different ways. In protistans, such as the amoeba, nitrogenous wastes simply diffuse across the cell membrane and out into the surrounding water.

However, since protoplasm is hypertonic to pond water, water constantly enters the body by osmosis, threatening to cause the organism to swell and rupture. (You may recall our earlier discussion of osmosis.) Some protistans must constantly expel water by the continual pumping of a contractile vacuole.

In the case of freshwater protists, then, the problems of metabolic waste and internal water regulation are solved by different mechanisms. In the animals, the two problems may be solved by the same mechanisms.

As an example of a single mechanism adjusting the body's level of both metabolic wastes and water content, consider the excretory system of the earthworm. Each segment of an earthworm has a pair of coiled tubes called *nephridia*, connecting the body cavity to the outside. The tubes opening inside the body cavity are rimmed with beating cilia that circulate the fluids there.

Capillaries lie tightly coiled around the outside of the nephridia, and as the fluid moves into and through the tube toward the outside, water, salts, and minerals are drawn back into the capillaries. The concentrated waste, then, is excreted through the external pore. The amount of water the animal excretes with the wastes (primarily urea and ammonia) depends on how much water has entered the body cavity. Worm urine, in case you've ever wondered, is very dilute, and the amount excreted each day equals about 60 percent of the worm's body weight.

The Human Kidney

Humans, as do the other mammals, have two kidneys (although we can live with one). These lie in the dorsal area (at the back) and extend slightly below the protective rib cage (which is one reason blows to the kidney area are so dangerous). Actually, they lie behind the membrane that lines the abdominal cavity. Each kidney contains about a million *nephrons*, each consisting of a *glomerulus* (a tightly convoluted blood vessel) a cuplike *Bowman's capsule* surrounding the glomerulus, and the connecting *tubules* leading from the capsule to the *collecting duct* (where urine collects on the way to the urinary bladder). The structure of these units is shown, along with the position of the kidney itself.

The basic mechanism of urine formation involves filtering all but the very large substances out of the blood and then adjusting the filtrate by reabsorbing substances needed by the body back into the blood, and by actively secreting some substances from the blood into the filtrate. Thus we see that there are three processes involved in urine formation: filtration, reabsorption, and secretion.

Let's see how this happens. First, the blood is filtered through the glomerulus into Bowman's capsule. The exit from the glomerulus is smaller than the entrance, so that blood is placed under high pressure as it enters the *artery*. As the blood wends its way through the tortuous route of the glomerulus, much of its fluids are forced out through the thin-walled vessels and into the cuplike Bowman's capsule. Most larger

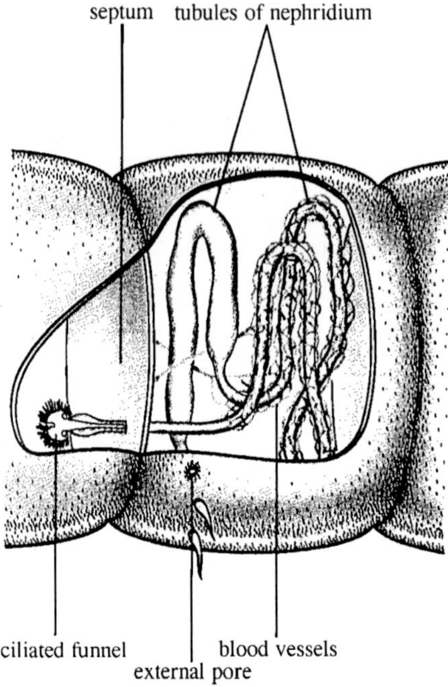

Figure 2.2 : Nephridium of an earthworm. Most segments boast a pair of nephridia.

particles, such as blood cells and most proteins, cannot pass through the glomerular walls.

The filtrate received by the Bowman's capsule contains a high concentration of waste products, but also water, salts, and nutrients. So, as the filtrate begins to move through the tubules on its journey to the urinary bladder, it passes through the twisted proximal convoluted tubule, down through the hairpin turn of the *loop of Henle*, up to the distal convoluted tubule, and on to the collecting ducts.

Blood vessels from the glomerulus head off the filtrate at the convoluted tubules and the loop of Henle. The blood vessels wind around the tubules and the loop and retrieve many of the usable products, both through diffusion and by active transport, allowing the urea and some water to continue on their way.

The remaining fluid in the tubules proceeds to a larger collecting tubule, and then to the *ureter*, which leads from each kidney to the *urinary bladder*. From the urinary bladder, the urine passes through a single opening, controlled by sphincter muscles, that leads into the *urethra* and on to the outside.

The Concentration of Urine

The conservation of water during urine formation is crucial. Although water conservation actually takes place primarily in the collecting ducts, it depends on the activities of the *loops of Henle*.

The principal role of the loop of *Henle* is to create a dense salt concentration in its surroundings, the kidney medulla. With a million *nephrons* participating, the salt concentration in the medulla becomes considerable.

A high salt concentration means a low water concentration much lower than the water concentration inside the nephron, so that a natural osmotic gradient forms. Simply stated, where salt goes, water will follow. But how does the loop accomplish this? The answer lies in its peculiar hairpin shape and some very capable cells in the ascending limb of the loop.

As the crude *filtrate* makes its way through the loop, cells in the ascending limb actively transport salt out of the filtrate. Much of the salt leaving the ascending limb moves across to the *descending limb*, it simply diffuses back into the loop (another example of a countercurrent exchange).

Table 1.2 : Urinary System

Strucutre	*Function*
Kidney	Filters blood and produces urine in nephron
Glomerulus	Filters blood
Bowman's capsule	Catches the filtrate
Proximal convoluted tubule	Selectively reabsorbs water, salts, nutrients
Loop of Henle	Secretes sodium chloride, concentrates urine
Distal convoluted tubule	Reabsorbs sodium, secretes H+, K+ and certain drugs
Collecting duct	Reabsorbs water under influence of ADH
Ureter	Carries urine to bladder
Bladder	Stores urine
Urethra	Eliminates urine

We see then, that the continuous cycling of salt in and out of the loop produces the necessary osmotic gradient. Further, active transport also moves some of the salt into the nearby capillary bed, thus extending

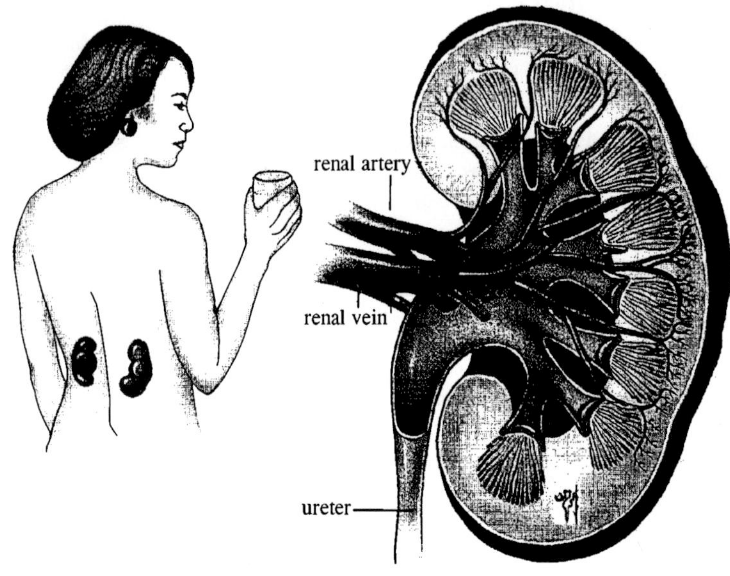

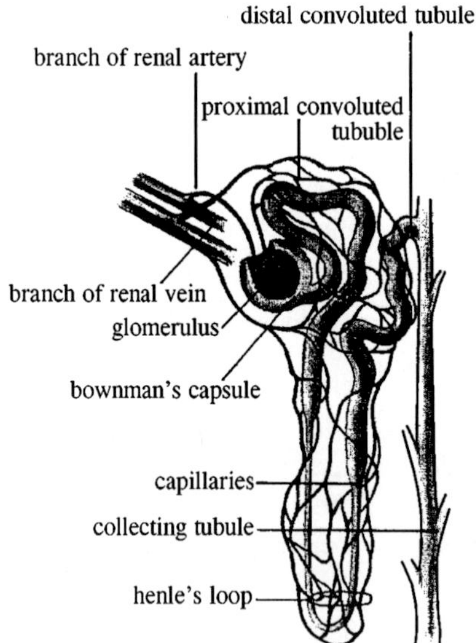

Figure 2.3 : The human kidney. Note the position of the kidneys in the body. The lower part actually extends below the protective rib cage. Also note the vast maze of blood vessels penetrating the kidney. Blood is brought into the kidney under considerable force, and many of its constituents are filtered through the glomeruli.

the gradient. As a result, water continually leaves the descending limb of the loop, moves through the salty medulla, and enters the surrounding capillaries.

Interestingly, the osmotic gradient we've been describing gets a boost in a seemingly odd way. Urea, which is concentrating in the collecting duct, moves out, thereby adding another solute to the salty medulla. It reenters the nephron at Henle's loop, returning to the collecting duct and thereby forming its own cycle. So urea, the primary nitrogenous waste, also plays a role in water retention.

Have you ever noticed how often your rowdy, beer-drinking friends must urinate once the evening gets underway? You may have heard them comment that more seems to be going out than was coming in. The next day they may complain of being thirsty. In your stern lecture to them you should say something about the diuretic effects of ethyl alcohol.

You will find them particularly interested when you say that the reason for their thirst is that reabsorption of water at the collecting ducts is controlled by an *antidiuretic hormone* (ADH) that is secreted by the posterior lobe of the pituitary in the brain. Go on to say that alcohol suppresses the secretion of this hormone, resulting in less water being reabsorbed from the collecting ducts. The urine thus becomes hypotonic, or more dilute than the body fluids, and the body actually becomes somewhat dehydrated.

Point out that, on the other hand, ADH secretion also decreases when you drink a great deal of water, since the osmotic concentration of the blood decreases (so drinking water can temporarily "thin" the blood). Drinking water, you can say, also results in the formation of a urine that is hypotonic to the blood. They will appreciate this information, especially early the next morning.

If your friends are so appreciative that they buy you a sailboat, you may be interested in another bit of practical physiology. If you discover, far at sea, that for some strange reason the boat sinks, you should know that a person on a life raft cannot get the water he needs by eating fish, contrary to popular rumor. The reason is that human urine cannot exceed a salt concentration higher than about 2.2 percent.

Fish fluids are not actually this concentrated, but fish are high in protein. This means that in order to get rid of the excess nitrogen, you would have to excrete a lot more water than you could get from eating the fish. Of course, you would do better eating fish than drinking seawater, since the salt concentration in seawater is about 3.5 percent.

Some shipwreck survivors claim that the spinal fluid of fish is a good supply of water, but all things considered, you would be better off to have remembered to take water along.

3

NUTRITION

This chapter combines two related topics: cellular metabolism and human nutrition. We discuss these topics together because a healthy diet can be planned only in terms of body needs. Body needs, in turn, depend on cell activities.

The functions we describe are basic to all organisms. They apply to brain cells and liver cells but also to bacteria and green plants. You will find that this chapter builds directly on the previous one. A review of cell structure and cell chemicals may help you understand the ideas we present here.

In order to live, cells must metabolise. That is to say, cells must transform nutrients into energy and into their own characteristic components. Cells need energy to move, to conduct bioelectric impulses, to accumulate nutrients, and to perform many other functions. Living is a dynamic process of continuous chemical activity.

Healthy cells ceaselessly adjust, repair, and replace themselves. Of course, doing these things means making new molecules, and that requires energy, too.

Considering what has just been said, we can see that there are really two aspects to metabolism: *degradation*, breaking down, and *synthesis*, building up. One drives the other. Degradation of nutrients provides energy and raw materials for synthetic reactions.

Some nutrients must be available in bulk amounts to supply the vast energy and raw material requirements of cells. Other nutrients are needed in much smaller quantities but are nonetheless essential because they cannot by synthesized from the major nutrients. For this reason, no single nutrient can sustain all the metabolic reactions of cells. In the next few pages, we will explore the topic of cellular metabolism in some detail. Then we will put this information to practical use when we discuss human nutrition in the latter part of the chapter.

EXTRACTING ENERGY FROM NUTRIENTS

In other Chapter, we discussed oxidation-reduction reactions as the chief way in which cells obtain energy from chemicals. The example we gave then was the oxidation of glucose.

$$\underset{\text{glucose}}{C_6H_{12}O_6} + \underset{\text{carbon dioxide}}{6O_2} \rightarrow \underset{\text{carbon dioxide}}{6CO_2} + \underset{\text{water}}{6H_2O} + \text{Energy}$$

This single-step reaction is what would occur if glucose was burned in air. As with other combustion reactions-exploding gasoline, for example—a great deal of heat energy is released all at once. Within cells glucose is degraded differently. High temperatures and sudden release of large amounts of energy are not compatible with life.

Cellular oxidation-reduction reactions occur in a piecemeal fashion so that energy is released slowly and in small, controllable amounts. In fact, cellular metabolism, whether degradative or synthetic, occurs by a progression of carefully controlled enzymatic steps.

Enzymes and Metabolic Control

If you have ever built a fire, you know that it is not a simple job. The logs must be arranged just so. And there must be kindling to produce sufficient heat to ignite the larger pieces of wood. Similarly, an electric spark is necessary to release energy from the gasoline in an automobile engine.

In a way, enzymes act as kindling for metabolic reactions. But instead of supplying energy, as kindling does, enzymes reduce the *activation energy* needed for a reaction.

A substance that increases the rate of a reaction by lowering the activation energy barrier is called a *catalyst*. Chemists have discovered a variety of catalysts that can speed their test tube reactions. Enzymes are biological catalysts. They speed up cell reactions that would otherwise occur only slowly -too slowly to support living systems at temperatures that permit life. Just like kindling, enzymes are effective in small doses. Unlike kindling, however, enzymes are not consumed in the reactions they promote. They can be used over and over again.

How Enzymes Do It

Enzymes are proteins, consisting of one or more long chains of

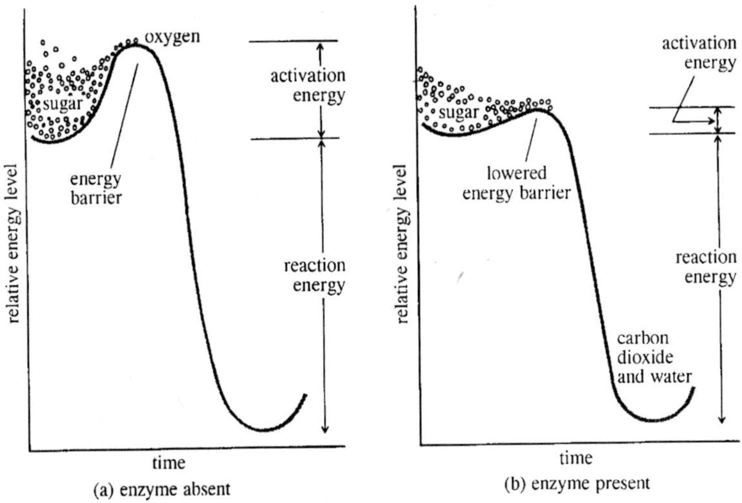

Figure 3.1 : Effect of an enzyme on activation energy.

amino acids. As with other proteins, multitudes of weak bonds between amino acids at different points cause the chains to fold and twist very precisely, so each enzyme has a unique structure. Most important, the arrangement of amino acid chains provides a surface where catalytic activity is centered.

Part of the surface of every enzyme is shaped into an *active site*. This place is where *substrates* (substances to be changed) bind to the enzyme. The active site conforms to the shape of substrate molecules. Although enzyme and substrate combine, the union is only temporary. Soon the substrate is converted into the *product*, which separates from the enzyme. This leaves the enzyme free to catalyze the reaction of still more substrate molecules.

A chemist might try to accelerate a test tube reaction by heating the contents of the tube. This may do the job, because at elevated temperatures molecules move about more rapidly and are much more likely to bump into one another and react. Just as important, fast-moving molecules frequently collide with sufficient force to cause chemical bonds to rupture or rearrange. Of course, not all collisions, not even all forceful ones, result in reactions. Reactions, as we learned in other Chapter of this book, occur only when they are energetically favourable. Nevertheless, even energetically favourable reactions will not occur unless the chemically reactive portions of reactant molecules come into contact.

There is probably no single explanation for how all enzymes work. As with ordinary chemical reactions, *enzymatic* ones usually involve more than one substance. Where there is more than one substrate, the affinity of the enzyme for the substrates effectively increases collisions between the reactants. In a cell, therefore, an *enzyme* sorts its *substrates* out of the mixture of substances found there.

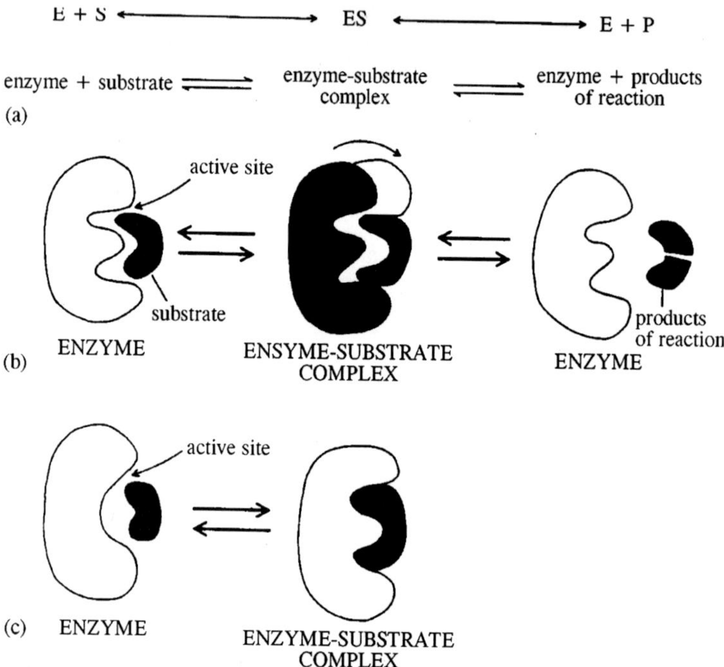

Figure 3.2 : Interaction of enzyme and substrate.

Furthermore, the active site is a perfect meeting place, because it permits the enzyme to hold the substrate *molecules* in positions that favour reaction between them.

Careful study of a few enzymes indicates that the binding of substrate to enzyme induces the enzyme to mold itself more closely to the substrate. Apparently the enzyme then proceeds to squeeze and strain the substrate molecule and weaken its bonds. Is it any wonder, then, that substrates are more reactive in the presence of their enzymes?

Considering how enzymes operate, we can now appreciate the importance of the numerous, though individually weak, bonds that shape an enzyme. If an enzyme were held in some rigid configuration by strong bonds, it would be *immobilised*. Effective enzyme action requires pliability. Because an enzyme is rather loosely shaped, it can easily mold itself to substrates.

The requirement that enzymes fit their substrates explains the specific nature of enzymes. There is no all-purpose enzyme. We have a specific enzyme for almost every metabolic reaction.

Enzyme Sensitivity

Because enzymes can be used over and over again, cells require only a limited number of each kind. Still, just like all tools, enzymes wear out and must eventually be replaced. When enzymes lose their unique shape and consequently their active site, they are said to be *denatured*. Denaturation may result from ordinary wear and tear or from various forms of environmental damage.

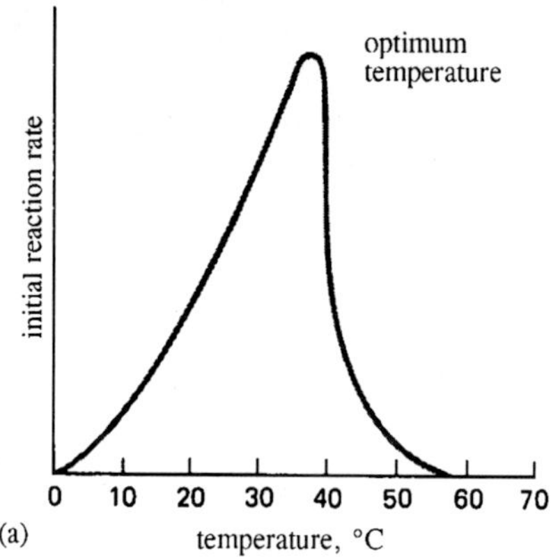

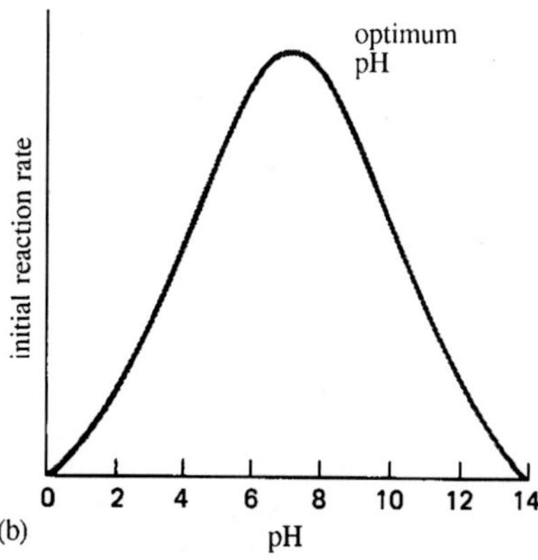

Figure 3.3: Effect of temperature and pH on enzymes.

Easy susceptibility to denaturation is the price proteins pay for their exceptional structural characteristics. The weak bonds so easily rearranged in the course of enzyme activity can be permanently disrupted by high temperatures. It is true, however, that a few enzymes are particularly resistant to heat, at least for short periods. Some examples are the enzymes that are obtained from cells and used as cleansing agents or as meat tenderizers.

To a great extent, the heat sensitivity of essential enzymes determines the maximum temperature an organism can tolerate. We take advantage of this fact when we use heat to destroy harmful "*germs*" in food or water. The temperature sensitivity of enzymes also explains why a high fever is so dangerous. Some human cells die quickly at temperatures above 42.2°C (108°F) because their enzymes "cook" or denature. Normal body temperature is 37°C (98.6°F).

Enzyme structure and function are also affected by acidity or alkalinity. Many enzymes seem to work best in a neutral environment that is neither acid nor alkaline. Others can function in stomach acid of about pH2, strong enough to burn a hole in this page.

For the most part, digestive enzymes are extracellular enzymes, secreted by cells to the outside. Inside a cell, numerous membranous compartments provide *mini-environments* with conditions appropriate for the function of the enzymes located there.

Many poisons are chemicals that react with enzymes and denature them. This explains the deadly effect of cyanide, the heavy metals lead and mercury, and certain other chemicals. When a poison such as mercury is taken by mouth, a common antidote is egg white. It must be administered shortly after the poison is ingested, however. In the stomach the poison reacts with the egg white protein much as it would react with enzyme protein.

In so doing, the poison becomes trapped in the precipitated, denatured egg white. A stomach pump must be used to remove the precipitate, or something must be given to cause vomiting. Otherwise the denatured egg white will eventually be digested and the poison released back into the system.

Inhibition can be Useful

Although we generally think of inhibition as undesirable, it is one means cells use to regulate their metabolism. Intracellular metabolism can be manipulated by subtle changes of pH. For instance, acid production in a cellular compartment may inhibit some enzymes but activate others. Perhaps a more dramatic kind of control, however, is the

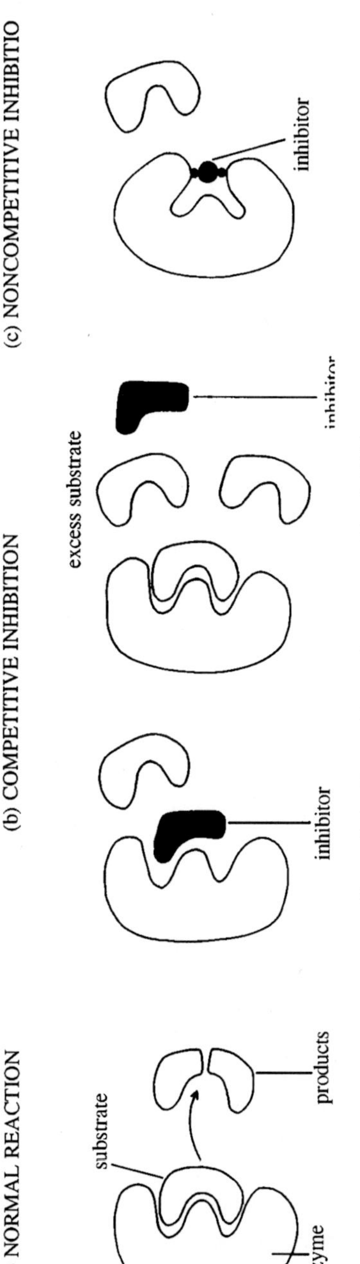

Figure 3.4 : Competitive and non-competitive inhibition.

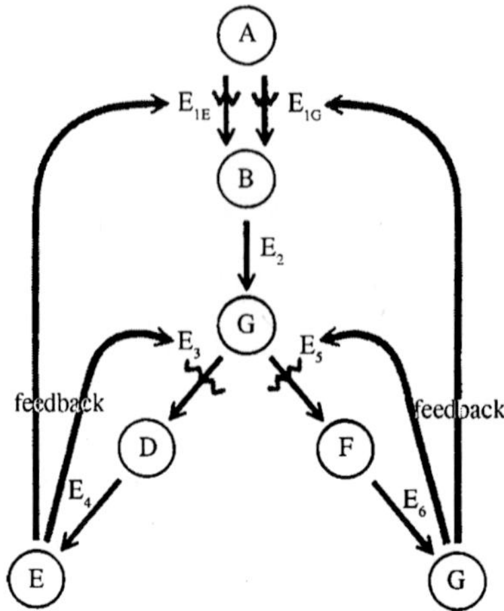

Figure 3.5 : Concerted feedback control.

phenomenon of *feedback regulation*. In this process, accumulation of the end product of an enzymatic sequence inhibits one or more key enzymes involved in its production.

Feedback regulation involves alteration in the shape of the affected enzyme. An enzyme under feed back control has a control site as well as an active site. When the end product of the reaction sequence begins to accumulate, it binds to the control site of the enzyme. This distorts the enzyme's shape, so the *substrate* can no longer gain access to the active site. As a consequence, the enzyme cannot work and the whole reaction sequence grinds to a halt.

So long as there is a need for the end product, it does not accumulate and the reaction sequence that produces it proceeds normally. But when the supply of product exceeds the demand, the sequence begins to slow down. Usually enzymes fairly early in the reaction sequence are stopped by feedback regulation. This is an efficient means of control since it prevents the wasteful accumulation of intermediates that would occur if the sequence of events was halted at a later point.

Eventually the backlog of end product will begin to disappear as it is used up by other metabolic reactions. At some point demand for the end product becomes so great that even those molecules bound to inhibited enzymes will be released. This permits the enzymes to function, thus turning on the reaction sequence once more.

Feedback regulation permits a cell to turn on or turn off selected chemical reactions. So you see, enzymes not only catalyze the chemical reactions of life, but regulate them as well!

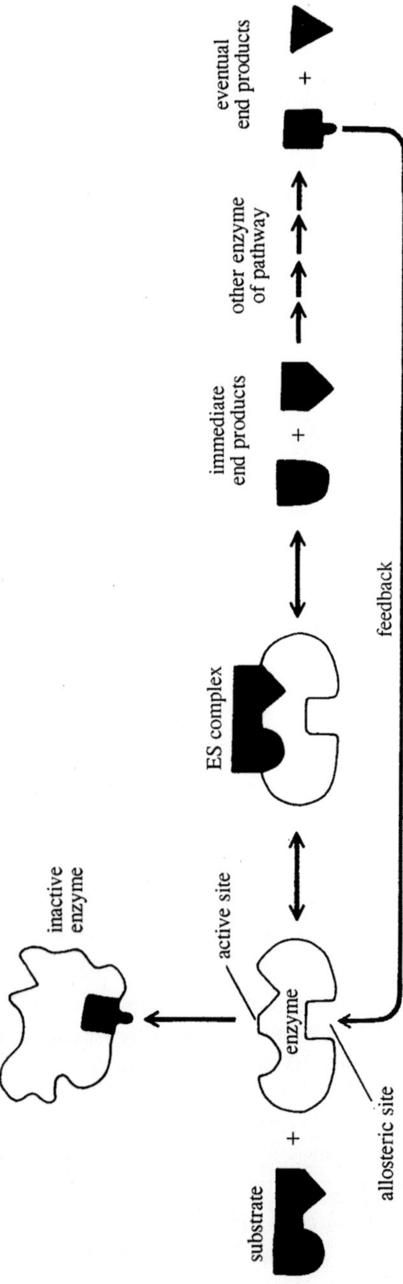

Figure 3.6 : How enzymes are controlled by feed back.

Enzymes and Energy Capture

At the beginning of this chapter we stressed the importance of the difference between combustion, in which energy is released "at a *single blow*," and biological oxidations. Well, we might also have mentioned that biological oxidations are not as slow as other kinds of oxidation, such as the rusting of metal. Enzymes cause biological oxidations to occur one step at a time, at just the right rate of speed, and in such a way that when energy is released, it can be captured and used to perform *cellular work*. We have already learned something about the kinds of reactions that yield energy, but how is energy captured?

Coupled Reactions

Earlier we mentioned that the most common type of biological oxidation is a *dehydrogenation*, whereby hydrogens (and their accompanying *electrons*) are removed from an organic compound, as shown below.

$$\underset{\substack{\text{H donor} \\ \text{(energy} \\ \text{source)}}}{AH_2} + \underset{\text{H acceptor}}{B} \rightarrow \underset{\substack{\text{oxidised} \\ \text{product}}}{A} + \underset{\substack{\text{reduced} \\ \text{product}}}{BH_2} + \text{Energy}$$

Although heat would be released if this reaction occurred in a test tube, inside a cell most of the energy of *dehydrogenation* reactions is not simply set free. Instead of being largely wasted as heat, it is transfe-rred to another compound, adenosine triphosphate, known as ATP. The participation of ATP is another unique aspect of biological oxidations.

Cells capture energy released in *biological oxidations* by making ATP. Since ATP formation requires energy, we say that the synthesis of ATP is coupled to biological oxidations, such as dehydrogenations. Enzymes accomplish the coupling. Energy lost when the bonds of nutrient molecules are broken is used to make the bonds of ATP, which is produced from adenosine diphosphate (ADP) and inorganic phosphate.

We can see the nature of so-called *coupled reactions* that produce ATP by summing up the two kinds of reactions we've been talking about: one energy-yielding, the other energy-requiring.

1. $AH_2 + B \xrightarrow{\text{enzyme 1}} A + BH_2 + \text{Energy}$

2. $ADP + P + \text{Energy} \xrightarrow{\text{enzyme 2}} ATP$

Overall: $AH_2 + B + ADP + P \rightarrow A + BH_2 + ATP$

Often such reactions are simplified by writing them as follows:

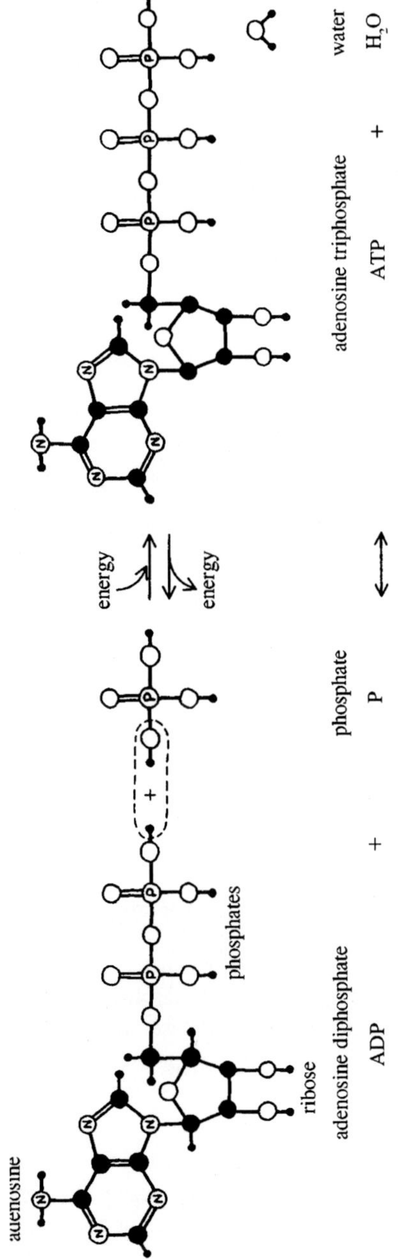

Figure 3.7 : ATP formation.

$$AH_2 + B \xrightarrow{\quad ADP \curvearrowright ATP \quad} A + BH_2$$

How ATP is Used

We don't expect the furnace that heats our home to supply the energy to run all the appliances and mow the lawn. On the other hand, this would not be an *unreasonable* expectation if the furnace powered an electric generator. Conversion of heat energy into electrical energy makes possible the performance of a greater variety of tasks. A cell may be compared to a *modern power plant* that produces *electricity* from coal, gas, or oil. Cells similarly convert energy from many chemically different nutrients into a single useful form, but instead of making electricity, they make ATP.

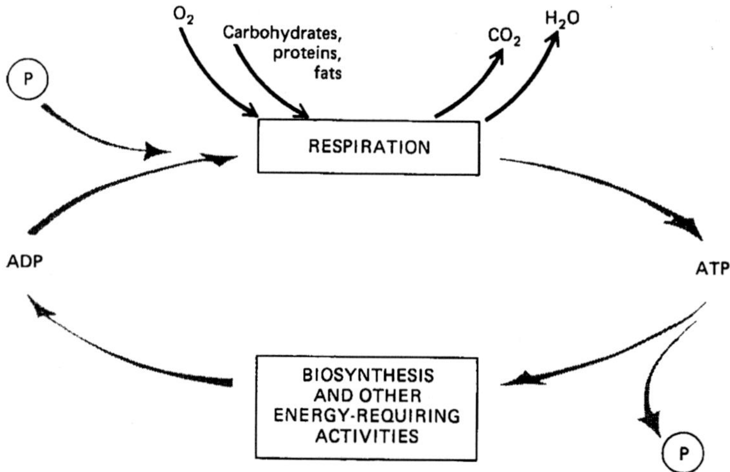

Figure 3.8 : The ADP-ATP.

The principal *energy-transfer compound* of cells, ATP has been called an "*energy currency.*" A cell can pay the energy price for its many operations by using ATP as a general power source. When ATP powers a cellular function, the ATP loses one of its phosphates and becomes ADP. ATP is later *regenerated* when food molecules are oxidised. The energy that is released from food is used to add *phosphate* to ADP.

The ADP-ATP cycle is illustrated in Figure elsewhere in this chpater. The cycle operates much like a rechargeable battery that provides a constant supply of electricity. However, not all the energy released by biological oxidations is harnessed in the form of ATP. Because all energy conversions are inefficient, some energy is always lost as heat. Part of this heat energy is used to maintain the body temperature.

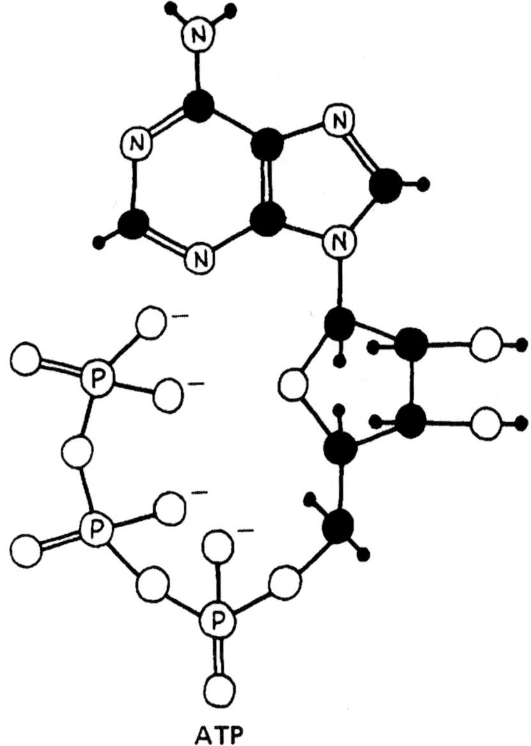

Figure 3.9 : The energy in ATP.

Before going further, let us stop to consider an important point about ATP. It is not an energy storage compound. Cells do not manufacture piles of ATP for later use. The chemical nature of ATP is such that it is extremely reactive. An ATP molecule is poised, like a spring, ready to give up its energy at the slightest provocation.

It just wouldn't be safe to try to store energy in such a volatile form. All could be lost by "*spontaneous combustion.*" Instead, cells make ATP continuously and use it immediately. Energy is stored by converting excess nutrients into such relatively stable substances as fats.

Every body cell makes the ATP it needs by oxidising nutrient molecules. These energy-rich substances are systematically degraded into smaller and smaller pieces, and the energy is transferred to ATP.

Not every metabolic step is an oxidation step. Some of the reactions are preparatory steps that make the capture of energy more efficient in the end. Eventually, however, only energy-poor waste products are left. Although all major types of food molecules can be oxidised, carbohydrates are especially important energy sources.

GENERATING ATP FROM CARBOHYDRATES

Before we can get energy from the food we eat, the food must be digested. Digestion does not actually release any biologically useful energy. It is merely the process by which food is converted into a form that can be absorbed into the body. Humans eat and di- r gest a variety of carbohydrates, but most individual 'L body cells are served only *glucose*. In other Chapter of this book we will describe how the body converts other carbohydrates into this simple sugar. For now, let us consider only how cells obtain energy from the glucose made available to them.

In cells, the breakdown of glucose to carbon dioxide and water requires something like two dozen different enzymatic steps. The process is often referred to as *cellular respiration*, because it involves the consumption of oxygen and the evolution of carbon dioxide. However, oxygen is not needed for the first ten reactions. Accordingly, cellular respiration can be divided into two stages. The first, *glycolysis*, is anaerobic, that is, does not require oxygen. Only the second stage of glucose metabolism is aerobic, or oxygen-requiring.

Stage I. Glycolysis occurs in the cytoplasm of a cell. In summary what happens is this:

$$\text{glucose} + 2\text{ADP} + 2\text{ phosphate} + 2\text{NAD} \rightarrow 2\text{ pyruvic acid} + 2\text{ATP} + 2\text{NADH}_2$$

Figure elsewhere in this chapter tells the full story. As you can see, the first few *glycolytic* reactions involve subtle changes in the glucose molecule. Note that two of the early steps are priming reactions that utilise ATP energy. These reactions prepare the glucose for the more drastic steps that lie ahead. They make ATP synthesis possible.

Eventually, the *six-carbon* sugar is cleaved into two pieces. Then each of the three-carbon fragments is partially oxidised. Here is an example of a biological oxidation that does not involve oxygen. The two three-carbon fragments are oxidised by being stripped of some of their hydrogens. These hydrogens carry with them a portion of the energy that was locked into the original glucose molecule. The enzyme that removes the hydrogens deposits them with a *hydrogen carrier* named NAD, a

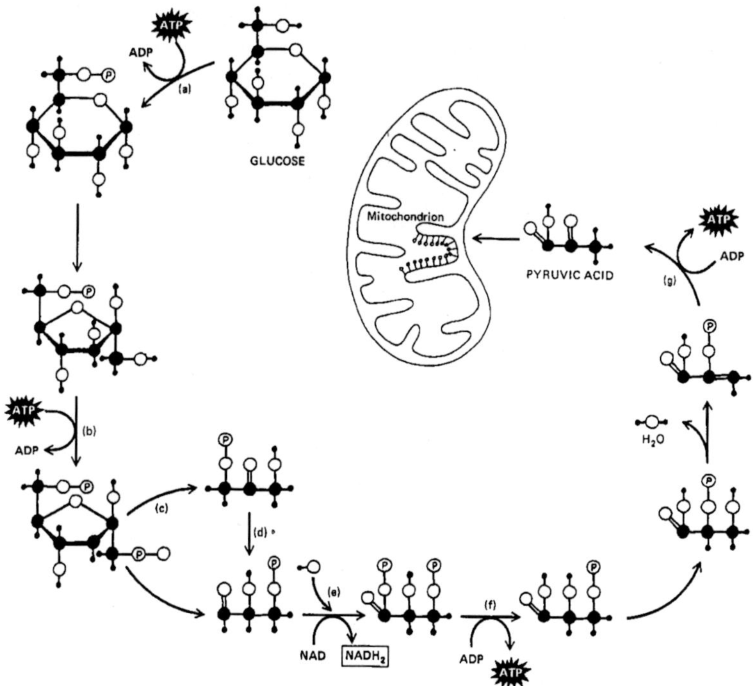

Figure 3.10 : Glycolysis.

substance that is derived from the vitamin niacin. The reaction occurs as follows:

$$NAD + 2H \rightarrow NADH_2$$

The oxidised sugar *fragments* have unstable structures. They quickly degenerate, giving up some of their energy by reacting with ADP to produce ATP. In the end, each of the three-carbon fragments has been converted into *pyruvic acid*. Note that again no oxygen has been utilised and no carbon dioxide has been produced.

Stage II. When there is an adequate supply of oxygen, the pyruvic acid produced in glycolysis can be oxidised to carbon dioxide and water. The overall result can be summarised as follows:

$$2 \text{ pyruvic acid} + 36ADP + 36P + 6O_2 \rightarrow$$
$$3CO_2 + 12H_2O + 36ATP$$

The process begins with the movement of pyruvic acid into the mitochondria.

The reactions that occur within the *mitochondria* are complicated but extremely efficient in extracting chemical energy from pyruvic acid. Almost 20 times more ATP is generated in the mitochondria than through glycolysis, which occurs in the surrounding cytoplasm. The reactions are collectively called the Krebs cycle or the metabolic mill.

Why the Krebs Cycle is a Metabolic Mill

As soon as pyruvic acid arrives at the interior of a mitochondrion, it is attacked by enzymes that first split off a carbon dioxide and then remove some energy-rich hydrogen atoms, passing them to waiting hydrogen carriers. The two-carbon acetic acid that remains is fed into the Krebs cycle *metabolic mill*. This cyclic enzymatic sequence is a busy oxidation factory. It degrades acetic acid into carbon dioxide and, in so doing, releases more hydrogens.

Acetic acid is drawn into the metabolic mill by reacting with a special acceptor found in the mitochondrion. As this complex is acted on by one and then another enzyme of the mill, more and more hydrogens are detached. Some of the hydrogens are passed to NAD, and others combine with a different hydrogen carrier, FP, which is a derivative of the vitamin riboflavin. In time, each of the two dehydrogenated acetic acid carbons is released as carbon dioxide.

And at one point during the degradations, enough energy is released to convert ADP to ATP. In the course of subsequent reactions, the acetic acid acceptor is regenerated, thus closing the cycle. The cycle recommences when the rejuvenated carrier picks up a new acetic acid fragment. Upon completion of each "turn" of the metabolic mill, one threecarbon pyruvic acid is oxidised to three molecules of carbon dioxide.

The Respiratory Chain

As you have probably noticed, oxygen is not directly involved in the oxidations of the *metabolic mill*. Nevertheless, oxygen must be present for the mill to operate. Oxygen acts as the *final acceptor* of the hydrogens that were only temporarily deposited with the hydrogen carriers. If these carriers are not relieved of their load in this way, the limited number of carrier molecules in a cell are all soon filled up, and energy-yielding oxidations abruptly cease.

By passing their hydrogens to oxygen, the carriers are again free to pick up more hydrogens and thereby keep respiration going. Water is the product of this reaction. Hydrogen carrier molecules do not pass the hydrogens they hold directly to oxygen. Instead, they feed them into the *respiratory chain*, a group of closely linked molecules packed into the neatly folded mitochondrial membranes. At least five different components are involved in the action of the respiratory chain. Of special importance are the *cytochromes*. These proteins are iron-containing pigments. They catalyze the last four steps of the respiratory chain.

The respiratory chain operates something like a bucket brigade. The energy-laden hydrogens are passed along the chain from one enzyme to another by means of a series of *oxidation-reduction* reactions. With each transfer a little energy is "*spilled.*" At several points in the chain enough energy is released to manufacture ATP. Finally, the energydrained hydrogens are given to oxygen, and water is formed. Most of the ATPs produced in the complete oxidation of glucose are synthesized in the *respiratory chain*.

Table 3.1 : ATP Yield from Glucose.

Stage of Respiration	*Number of ATP*
Glycolysis	2
Mitochondrial oxidations	
Krebs metabolic mill	2
Respiratory chain	34
Total (per glucose molecule)	38

Chemiosmotic ATP Synthesis

For many years biologists have been puzzled by how the energy "*spilled*" during mitochondrial oxidation-reduction reactions is captured to make ATP. The currently popular theory, the *chemiosmotic theory*, proposes that ATP synthesis is driven by a proton gradient created during operation of the respiratory chain.

A crucial property of many components of the respiratory chain is that they can carry electrons but not protons. You recall that biological oxidations usually involve removal of hydrogen atoms, and that hydrogen atoms consist of one electron and one proton. So, although hydrogens from glucose are fed into the respiratory chain, only electrons can travel the full length of the chain; their *companion protons* are scuttled along the way.

The *mystery* of the scuttled protons has always been heightened by the knowledge that they must finally be regained to make water. After all, water consists of two complete hydrogen atoms and one oxygen atom. The question has been: What are the protons doing in between? To answer that question, we need to know a little more about the structure of mitochondria.

Mitochondria have two membranes, but only the inner membrane is selectively permeable. And it is the inner membrane that contains the apparatus for making ATP. The inner membrane is constructed so as to create a proton gradient. Hydrogen carriers pass hydrogen atoms to the first member of the respiratory chain. This component then expels the protons outside the membrane and gives only the electrons to the next member of the chain.

Because the mitochondrial membrane is selectively permeable, the scuttled protons are segregated from the mitochondrial matrix. Thus the actions of the respiratory chain create a proton gradient in

which protons are accumulated on one side of the membrane. As the number of protons outside the inner membrane grows, that is, as the gradient grows, certain patches on the outer surface of the membrane become sensitized to the high level of protons.

These regions are associated with the *respiratory knobs* that line the mitochondrial cristae. At critical proton concentrations, the crowded protons force their way back through the membrane like a rush of water through a crack in a dike. The energy of this sudden surge of protons is what drives ATP synthesis.

Nearly all the oxygen taken up by a cell is consumed by mitochondrial respiratory chain oxidations. Red blood cells and other cells that lack mitochondria cannot use oxygen at all. Such cells are obliged to function anaerobically. The same is true of cells that are deprived of oxygen.

When There isn't Enough Oxygen to Go Around

In the absence of oxygen, that is, under anaerobic conditions, mitochondria cannot generate ATP, because there is no final electron acceptor. Without oxygen most body cells are deprived of their primary source of usable energy. Some cells, brain cells in particular, suffer serious damage if there is even a brief scarcity of oxygen. Others cope, at least for a while.

In humans, oxygen shortages occur during heavy exertion, such as running, when the circulation is not adequate to meet the oxygen demands of the muscles. Under these circumstances the pyruvic acid that cannot be oxidised by the mitochondria is transformed into *lactic acid*.

Under anaerobic conditions even glycolysis will grind to a halt unless some hydrogen acceptor is present to unload hydrogens from $NADH_2$. If the $NADH_2$ molecules were allowed to remain "*filled up*" because of the anaerobic condition, eventually there would be no NAD available to receive hydrogens, and glucose oxidation would come to an end. This is prevented when the hydrogens of $NADH_2$ are unloaded onto pyruvic acid, which is turned into lactic acid. Lactic acid is formed because pyruvic acid acts as a hydrogen acceptor in the absence of oxygen, and NAD molecules are then free to load up again.

As it happens, lactic acid is somewhat toxic. Humans can tolerate only a limited amount of lactic acid before discomfort requires a reduction in energy consumption. We become fatigued. The lactic acid dilates surface blood vessels, accounting in part for the flushed face that accompanies heavy exertion. Eventually exertion must cease because the body can tolerate no more lactic acid. The body can go into *oxygen debt* only so far.

When oxygen again becomes available, the lactic acid is converted into harmless compounds. The liver transforms most of the lactic acid into glycogen. The remainder of the pyruvic acid is immediately respired through the *metabolic mill*. The oxidation of so much pyruvic acid clearly produces a large amount of ATP. In addition, a great deal of

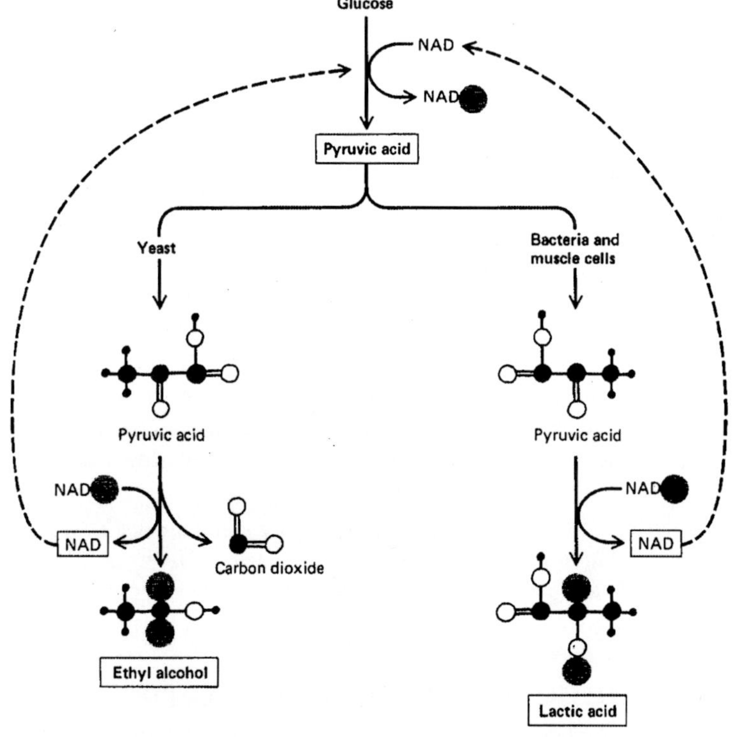

Figure 3.11 : Two fermentations.

heat is released, accounting for the surge of warmth we feel after the exertion is over.

There are some organisms that, unlike humans, are able to exist indefinitely in the total absence of oxygen. In these organisms glucose degradation is restricted to glycolysis. The pyruvic acid produced from glucose becomes the final hydrogen acceptor and is thereby converted into lactic acid. The souring of milk and certain other foods results from lactic acid produced by bacteria growing in the absence of oxygen. This process is called *fermentation*, but it is no different from what occurs in oxygenless muscle tissue.

A more familiar fermentation is the production of alcohol by yeast cells growing on grain or fruit under anaerobic conditions. Instead of forming lactic acid from pyruvic acid, yeasts split pyruvic acid into two parts, adding hydrogens from $NADH_2$ to one of them. In the end, ethyl alcohol and carbon dioxide are formed. The bubbles we associate with many *fermented beverages* are bubbles of carbon dioxide gas. So are the bubbles that make bread rise.

Generating ATP from Fats and Proteins

The metabolic mill is a versatile oxidation factory. Not only carbohydrates but most digestion products from proteins or fatty foods enter the mill at one point or another and are oxidised. To illustrate, let us consider the use of fats, which the body digests into *glycerol* and *fatty acids*. Glycerol is a three-carbon compound that is readily converted into *pyruvic acid* and respired.

The long fatty acid chains (16-18 carbons) are fragmented into two-carbon acetic acid units, which are also processed by the metabolic mill. Getting energy from proteins is more complicated, because the digestion of proteins yields 20 different kinds of amino acids. However, each amino acid is ultimately broken down to smaller pieces that can be oxidised by the enzymes of the metabolic mill.

Because the amino portion of every amino acid contains nitrogen, complete oxidation of proteins produces ammonia (NH_3) in addition to carbon dioxide and water. Sugars other than glucose are also metabolised. Thus all the major categories of human foods contain energy and can be oxidised to release energy.

NUTRITION, DIET, AND HEALTH

Earlier we mentioned that from the standpoint of nutrition, humans are classified as *heterotrophs*. Organisms as diverse as yeasts and *term-*

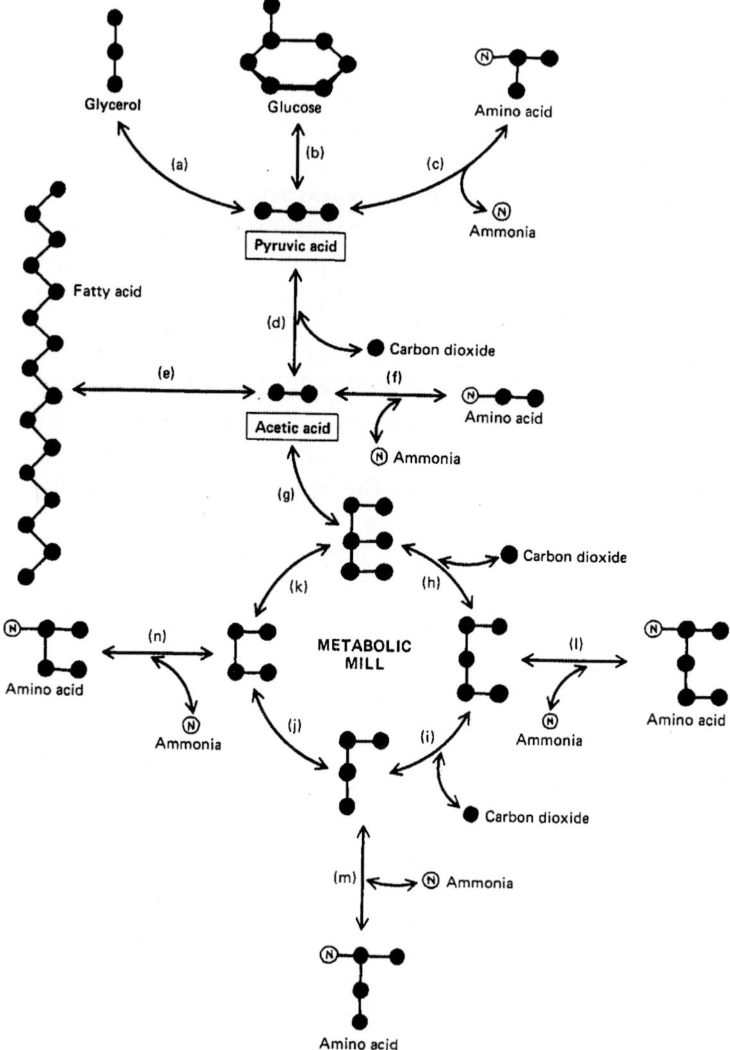

Figure 3.12 : All roads lead to the mill.

ites are heterotrophs, too, but we cannot survive indefinitely on the same diets that yeasts and termites eat. The food we eat must be in forms that our bodies can use and must include the proper quantities of particular *nutrients*. Although we can obtain energy from carbohydrates, proteins, or fats, our diet must supply amino acids for protein synthesis and small amounts of *vitamins*, *minerals*, and certain *fatty acids*.

Major Dietary Constituents: Form and Function

The bulk of the human diet is oxidised to obtain energy. In the United States today, carbohydrates provide 45 percent of an average individual's energy needs, another 40 percent comes from fats, and the remainder comes from protein. It apparently makes no difference which nutrients supply energy so long as the use of proteins for energy does not rob the body of its supply of amino acids.

Human energy needs vary with activity. Even at rest a minimum amount of energy is required to maintain the body. This includes energy for internal muscular movements, such as contraction of the heart, energy for operation of the nervous system, and energy for the synthesis of molecules to replace those that wear out.

By means of the instrument described in Figure elsewhere in this chapter, the caloric values of many foods have been determined. Of all the major food constituents, fats have been shown to have the highest caloric content: 9300 cal/gram. This may be compared with 4100 cal/gram for both *carbohydrates and proteins*. Keep in mind, however, that although energy is measured as heat, organisms do not use heat to perform most biological work.

The heat produced when food is burned in a combustion chamber is only a reflection of the amount of ATP energy that an organism would obtain from the food if it was eaten, digested, absorbed, and metabolised.

The amount of energy needed to satisfy the basal or resting requirements of a human depends on age, sex, and size of the individual. The average daily requirement for simple maintenance is 1500-2000 kilo calories. Anywhere from 500 to 4000 more may be needed for physical activity and for maintenance of body temperature in a cold environment. A person doing heavy labor may need more than twice as much energy as a sedentary business executive.

Common Denominators

Just as carbohydrates, fats, and proteins can all serve as energy sources, so they are to some extent interconvertible. This is possible because the metabolic mill is reversible. Not only do substances enter the mill to be oxidised, but mill intermediates can leave the cycle and be used in the manufacture of cellular building blocks. Thus glucose and proteins can be converted into fat. Similarly, fats and proteins can be used to synthesize glucose.

Conversion of glucose or fat into certain amino acids is possible but only if there is an adequate supply of amino groups. Normally we acquire these by eating protein and transferring amino groups from the constituent amino acids to metabolic mill components to synthesize other amino acids. Some important amino acids cannot be synthesized and must be eaten in the diet.

Building Blocks for Growth and Repair

Although proteins can serve as an energy source, they are much more important as raw material for growth and repair of body tissues. Protein is the principle *organic component* of the body. Human proteins contain 20 different amino acids, of which we can synthesize only ten. Those that we cannot synthesize are the *essential amino acids* and must be present in our diet. Consequently, we must eat enough protein to supply us with these amino acids.

A strictly protein diet must provide enough protein to meet all energy needs and the need for essential amino acids as well. On the other hand, if we eat only enough protein for normal growth and repair but insufficient carbohydrate or fat to supply energy, some of the precious protein will be oxidised for that purpose. The resulting shortage of amino acids will result in protein deficiencies that *impair health*.

Because various proteins differ in their content of essential amino acids, not all foods are adequate sources of raw material for synthesis of human proteins. Meat and such animal products as milk and eggs contain almost the same ratio of essential amino acids as do human tissue. Unfortunately, the same is not true of plant proteins.

Some plant foods are markedly deficient in one or more essential amino acids. For example, grains, such as wheat, rye, barley, oats, rice, and corn, contain little *lysine*, *isoleucine*, and *tryptophan*. However, most legumes, including beans and soybeans, have large amounts of these amino acids, but are low in *methionine* and *cystine*. Leafy green vegetables have a good balance of all the essential amino acids except methionine.

People who rely mainly on plants as a source of protein can receive an adequate assortment of amino acids only by combining proteins from several plant sources. Mexicans, for whom beans and corn or beans and rice are dietary staples, are among the many peoples who have evolved *nutritionally* sound mixtures of complementary foods.

There is convincing evidence to indicate that humans cannot synthesize certain unsaturated fatty acids needed to form some body structures. Fortunately, these *essential fatty acids* are present in nearly all foods and the amounts needed are so minute that deficiencies seldom occur.

Vitamins: Essential in Small Quantities

In comparison with their need for carbohydrates, fats, and proteins, our cells require only tiny amounts of vitamins. Largely for that reason, the importance of such compounds remained unknown until 1911. The term "vitamin" stresses their vital or essential nature. Vitamins are small organic molecules that ordinarily cannot be synthesized in sufficient quantity to meet body needs.

Therefore they must be provided in the diet. Vitamins do not serve as building blocks, nor are they energy sources. Each has a highly specialised function. A number are the principal ingredients for the enzyme helpers we call *coenzymes*. Coenzymes usually act as carrier molecules; they pick up chemical groups from one enzyme and pass them to another.

Although the biochemical roles of many vitamins are established, there is still controversy over the functions of others and over the amounts essential for optimal health. Many obstacles lie in the path of clear-cut determinations of human nutritional needs. Most important, ethical considerations limit human experimentation.

But scientists can establish absolute human requirements only by studying people. Some highlights concerning well-known vitamins appear in the next paragraphs. Table elsewhere in this chapter is a more comprehensive list of vitamins important for human health.

Scurvy, Colds, and Vitamin C

In the seventeenth century it was discovered that an ounce or so of lime juice daily would prevent the symptoms of scurvy among seamen; this led to the nickname "*limey*" for British sailors. The active ingredient in citrus juice turned out to be *ascorbic acid*, also known as *vitamin C*. Just 10 mg/day will alleviate the poor healing of wounds, tender gums, and bleeding that characterise *scurvy*.

There is still much to be learned about the biological importance of ascorbic acid. It is thought to be involved in oxidation reactions in cells, but the exact role is unclear. More specifically, vitamin C is required for the formation of collagen, the fibrous protein that holds tissues together. Scurvy symptoms result, at least in part, from loosening of the tissue in the absence of this vitamin.

There is some evidence, all of it controversial, that vitamin C can affect heart disease, colds, and even *cancer*. *Ascorbic acid* may be involved in cholesterol metabolism and thus in heart disease. (The relationship between *cholesterol* and heart attacks will be discussed in other Chapter.) Although some studies indicate that ascorbic acid cannot prevent colds, other data suggest that sufficient vitamin C may shorten the duration of a cold and lessen the symptoms. And although vitamin C may speed processes that rid the body of some cancer-causing chemicals, it may slow removal of others.

Because so many foods contain little or no vitamin C, we note its presence in substantial quantities in Brussels sprouts, mustard greens, and other members of the cabbage family. Probably these were important antiscurvy food for northerners before trade

brought oranges, tomatoes, and peppers, all rich in vitamin C. A high vitamin C content probably explains early use of such weed plants as pokeberry shoots, dock, and lambsquarter for "spring greens." Vitamin C breaks down *spontaneously* under some conditions. Consequently, stored or cooked products may contain less *vitamin C* than fresh foods. This is just one example of how manipulation of foods can reduce their nutritional value.

Thiamine (Vitamin B_1): a coenzyme discarded in milling

Minor thiamine deficiencies cause loss of appetite and weight. If prolonged, thiamine deficiency leads to degeneration of nerves and, in the extreme, heart failure. *Beri-beri*, as this condition is called, was once a serious *affliction* in the Orient, where rice is the staple food. The problem is that when rice is

polished, the tough seed coats that contain thiamine are removed. A diet high in polished rice can lead to beri-beri unless the rice is enriched with vitamin B_1. A similar problem involves wheat flour.

A few generations ago all wheat bread was made with whole flour. Then the development of milling techniques led to the introduction of white flour. Unfortunately, 90 percent of the thiamine is discarded in the milling. Federal law requires that flour and bread be "*enriched*" by addition of vitamins to at least partially replace those lost in milling. But it is *ironic* that the additional labor, energy, and expense required to produce refined, enriched flour result in a *nutritionally* poorer product than our *greatgrandparents* ate.

Thiamine is so widespread in foods that deficiencies occur most often in individuals who rely on highly refined foods or on a very limited variety of nutrients. Some alcoholics fall into the latter category. They may satisfy most of their energy requirements with *alcohol* and eat very little food containing vitamins. Not surprisingly, many of the *physical symptoms* associated with severe *alcoholism* accompanied by malnutrition are relieved by *thiamine therapy*.

Table 3.2 : Vitamins.

Vitamin	*Name*	**Some Deficiency** *Symptoms*	*Some Sources*
A	carotene	dry, flaky skin; night blindness	green or yellow vegetables, fruits, egg yolk, fishliver oil
B-complex	thiamine (B_1)	beri-beri, paralysis, heart failure, mental confusion	yeast, liver, pork, nuts, whole grains
	riboflavin (B_2)	cataracts, cracked lips and tongue, poor growth	dairy products, yeast, eggs, whole grains
	niacin (B_3)	pellagra, irritability, skin lesions, abdominal pain	meat, yeast, whole grains
	pyridoxine (B_6)	inflamed skin, convulsions	fish, meat, whole grains, fresh vegetables
	cyanocobalamin (B_{12})	anemia	brain, kidney, liver, other meats
	biotin	inflamed skin and eyes, hair loss	liver, eggs, fresh vegetables
	folic acid	anemia	leafy vegetables, liver
	pantothenic acid	numbness of hands and feet, depressed resistance to infection	almost all food
C	ascorbic acid	scurvy, inability to form connective tissues	citrus fruits, tomatoes
D	calciferol and other compounds	rickets, defective bone	dairy products, eggs, fish oils

Our bodies use thiamine to make one of the *coenzymes* involved in the oxidation of pyruvic acid during cellular respiration. Without thiamine, glucose oxidation cannot be completed, and *pyruvic* and *lactic acids* accumulate. The poisonous effect of these acids and the decreased energy production because of incomplete glucose oxidation cause the symptoms of thiamine-deficiency disease.

Pellagra, Poverty, and Niacin

Thiamine isn't the only vitamin that acts as a coenzyme in energy metabolism. Niacin, another member of the B complex, forms part of NAD, the hydrogen carrier used in glycolysis and the metabolic mill. This important role of niacin is indicated by the dire symptoms of *pellagra*, a condition that develops in its absence. *Mild deficiencies* produce inflammation of the skin and the digestive tract, but in its severest form pellagra involves mental *aberrations* and causes death. Remarkably, the *nervousness*, *insomnia*, *irritability*, *suspiciousness*, *hallucinations*, and depression that characterise a severe case of pellagra disappear after only two days of niacin therapy.

Like several other vitamins, *niacin* is widespread in organisms, and deficiencies develop only from unusual diets. Often pellagra can be traced to a diet of corn supplemented with little else. Until the 1930s pellagra was common among the poor of the American South, for whom cornbread was the staple and who could not afford meat, vegetables, or other cereals. Ordinarily the body absorbs some of the niacin that *intestinal bacteria* make from the amino acid *tryptophan*. But corn contains limited tryptophan, as well as little *niacin*. This situation points out the importance of a balanced diet containing a variety of foods.

Vitamin A Conversions

Not only does the body convert vitamins into key molecules, but it can make some vitamins from other substances. In fact, the definition of certain vitamins is somewhat hazy. Vitamin A is a good example. Although it is available in some animal products, such as liver, milk, and egg yolks, we need not eat vitamin A as such.

Instead the body can convert *carotenes*, a widespread group of plant pigments, into vitamin A. Carotenes are abundant in green vegetables, including members of the cabbage family and the "weed greens" mentioned as vitamin C sources. It is *carotenes* that colour yellow and red fruits and vegetables.

Among those particularly rich in carotenes are carrots, sweet potatoes, tomatoes, apricots, and beets. This is one reason for the nutritional rule about eating one yellow (or red) vegetable in addition to a green vegetable every day. Vitamin A apparently has a variety of functions. One use is as a constituent of *rhodopsin*, an eye pigment necessary for vision in dim light. With inadequate vitamin A there is inadequate *rhodopsin*, and the eye becomes unresponsive to small amounts of light. This symptom of vitamin A deficiency is sometimes called "*night blindness.*"

Severe shortages of vitamin A lead to increased formation of *keratin*, a fibrous protein normally present in the skin. When vitamin A deficiency causes keratin to be made in the delicate coverings of the eyeball and in the tear gland, these tissues become dry and hard, and blindness can result. *Keratinization* of the lining of the lungs predisposes people to pneumonia and other respiratory infections. In some developing countries vitamin A deficiency is a major cause of childhood blindness and death.

Vitamin D: the Sunshine Vitamin

Sunlight transforms certain plant and animal molecules into vitamin D. In fact, the *ultraviolet light* of sunshine converts a cholesterol-like substance of the skin into vitamin D. Dietary sources of this vitamin include butter, milk, egg yolks, and fish oils, such as *cod liver oil*. In addition, many natural foods are fortified with vitamin D. Often such foods carry the label "*irradiated ergosterol added.*"

Ergosterol is a cholesterol derivative extracted from yeast. It is added to food, and the food is then exposed to ultraviolet rays, which convert ergosterol to vitamin D. Milk contains a substance similar to ergosterol; as a result, irradiation of milk serves to enrich its vitamin D content.

People who live in tropical or subtropical areas rarely suffer from inadequate vitamin D. In places where sunlight is limited, some vitamin D must be consumed. This is particularly true in regions toward the poles, where days are short much of the year and sunlight is reduced. In fact, there is a possibility that the very light skin of Scandinavian peoples is an adaptation to take advantage of the available ultraviolet radiations of the far north. Light skin would filter out a minimum of the valuable rays that produce vitamin D.

Vitamin D regulates the use of calcium and phosphorus by the body. It does so by stimulating intestinal cells to absorb these minerals from the food we eat. Vitamin D also controls the deposition of calcium and phosphorus by bone cells. Lack of vitamin D may cause *rickets*, a disease characterised by *malformation* of growing bones. Although adults need less vitamin D than children do, chronic deficiencies may lead to localised softening of bone even in adults. Too much vitamin D can be harmful. One effect is calcification or hardening of normally soft tissues. For example, excess vitamin D can cause minerals to accumulate in the kidney, impairing its function. It is quite likely that the dark skin of some races evolved as protection against excessive vitamin D production. Dark skin is also a protection against skin cancer, which may be caused by overexposure to ultraviolet radiation.

Minerals: Inorganic Nutrients

Inorganic substances are normal components of cells and must be present in the proper concentration in the fluids around cells. L' Indeed, cells expend considerable energy moving, concentrating, and ejecting mineral ions.

How Cells Use Minerals

Just as vitamins serve as coenzymes, minerals sometimes act as enzyme helpers. Many enzymes can function only in a specific ionic

Table 3.3 : Some Elements Important in Mineral Nutrition.

Element	*Chemical Symbol*	*Use in the Body*
*Calcium	Ca	bone structure, enzyme function
*Chlorine	Cl	nerve and muscle function
Chromium	Cr	insulin function
Cobalt	Co	enzyme function
Copper	Cu	essential for some oxidative enzymes
Fluorine	F	strength of teeth and bone
Iodine	I	thyroid hormone structure
Iron	Fe	hemoglobin and cytochrome structure
Magnesium	Mg	enzyme function, bone structure
Manganese	Mn	enyzme function
Phosphorus	P	bone structure; found in many organic molecules, including ATP and nucleic acids
Potassium	K	nerve and muscle function
Selenium	Se	liver function
Sodium	Na	nerve and muscle function, absorption of nutrients
Zinc	Zn	enzyme function

environment. For example, *calcium* ions are necessary for a crucial step in blood clotting. Minerals also serve to activate various processes. Inside muscle cells, calcium is concentrated in *membranous* compartments and released as the final step in a chain of messages that lead to contraction.

Many mineral elements become parts of organic molecules. Probably most readers know that *iron* is necessary for healthy blood. The reason is that hemoglobin, the molecule that carries oxygen in red blood cells, contains iron. And recall that iron is a component of the cytochromes of the mitochondrial respiratory chain. *Phosphorus* is another element needed to manufacture organic molecules. As we have seen, ADP becomes highly charged with energy when it adds a third phosphate to form ATP.

The thyroid gland in the neck incorporates *iodine* into a hormone it secretes. Through secretion of this hormone the thyroid gland is able to regulate cellular respiration. Iodine deficiencies result in lower levels of the thyroid hormone and thus lowered metabolism and even mental dulling. Severe deficiencies during pregnancy result in drastic mental retardation in the offspring. These children, known as *cretins*, are *hopelessly handicapped intellectually*.

Other symptoms of iodine deficiency include abnormal growth of the thyroid itself. Through a feedback mechanism, *inadequate hormone* production stimulates increased size of the gland, which in turn increases hormone production if iodine is present. But in the absence of iodine the growth is futile and results only in an enlarged thyroid that protrudes in the front of the neck as a *goiter*.

Bone as a Special Mineral Store

Cells deposit calcium and phosphorus around themselves in the course of bone development. This process makes bone hard, of course, but it provides more than skeletal support. Bone serves as a reservoir of *calcium* and *phosphorus* from which the living cells extract and circulate these minerals as they are needed elsewhere in the body.

This *dynamic equilibrium* between bone and the rest of the body ensures adequate calcium and phosphorus when there are temporary shortages in the diet. Problems develop when prolonged dietary deficiencies weaken bone by draining away the minerals. Teeth contain similar mineral deposits and also participate in this exchange.

Because of the need of calcium and phosphorus to form bones and teeth, infants need *tremendous amounts* of these minerals if they are to grow normally. Usually the need is met by the high mineral content of milk. However, milk production makes a large demand on the mother's body. Nursing mothers must eat well in order to maintain their own health, because they are obliged to supply calcium and phosphorus, even at the expense of withdrawing materials from their own teeth and bones. This drain starts during pregnancy while the baby is growing in the uterus.

As important as calcium and phosphorus are to teeth and bones, the crystals there should also con- . tain traces of other minerals, particularly *fluorine*. The incorporation of fluorine into the calcium *phosphate crystal* dramatically increases the strength of the crystal. As a matter of fact, individuals living in areas where this trace element is present in the water have fewer dental cavities than do those living in areas where the fluoride level is extremely low.

Mineral Sources

All cells, whether from plants or animals, have similar mineral requirements. And most organisms use them in about the same proportions. Thus a diet adequate in other respects supplies all the minerals we *ordinarily* need. Mineral deficiencies largely involve elements that are usable only in specific forms or that we absorb poorly. Important examples are calcium and iron.

We have already mentioned the importance of vitamin D to proper absorption and utilisation of calcium and phosphorus. Although the cause is uncertain, calcium absorption varies with the kind of food eaten. For instance, despite the fact that cow's milk contains four times more calcium than human milk does, children do not absorb calcium as readily from cow's milk as they do from human milk. Therefore infants drinking cow's milk have greater needs for vitamin D.

The form of iron we eat makes 'a large difference in whether or not it is absorbed. The environment of the digestive tract is also important. Inorganic *ferrous iron*, which carries two positive charges, is the easiest to absorb. Acid in the stomach helps convert other inorganic iron into the ferrous form. On the other hand, a high concentration of calcium or phosphorus in the diet reduces iron absorption. And unlikely as it seems, iron found in organic molecules is poorly absorbed. Some organic molecules in food tend to combine with inorganic iron and make it less absorbable.

Of course, iron deficiencies are not due totally to poor absorption. Some diets are inherently low in iron. Milk contains little iron, and babies maintained too long on an unsupplemented milk diet become *anemic*, or low in hemoglobin. Iron-deficiency anemias affect children at a rate as high as one in every three children between the ages of 4 and 24 months in the United States.

Iron-deficiency anemias also appear in individuals with chronic blood loss. The blood loss of *hookworm* infestations can cause anemia. So can *menstruation* in otherwise healthy women who do not consume adequate iron. In fact, iron-deficiency anemias are distressingly common among women of *reproductive age*. Persistent dieting can further aggravate this problem by reducing the amount of iron consumed.

Distribution of Trace Elements

Some elements are needed in quite small amounts by organisms. These *trace elements* are often rare or scattered unevenly through the biosphere. We have already mentioned that local deficiencies of fluorine have adverse effects on tooth structure.

The fluorine content of water ordinarily reflects the amount of this trace element in the surrounding soil and rock. Some communities now add minute amounts of sodium fluoride to their water supplies to ensure better tooth development and reduce cavities.

Controversy surrounds this practice, partly because larger doses of fluorine are poisonous, and even small excesses cause defective bone crystals. Another reason is that some people object to having no personal control over the supplementation.

Iodine is also a trace element. Although iodine is rare on land, it is abundant in the ocean. Soil iodine comes almost entirely from particles thrown into the air by ocean spray and carried worldwide by the wind. The iodine falls out of the air, but of course, coastal areas receive more than do inland regions.

Although it plays no known role in plants, iodine, as well as many other trace elements, is absorbed by roots and distributed throughout the plant. Then iodine is carried through the food chain by animals that eat the plants. Naturally sea foods contain more iodine than do those grown on the land. Likewise foods grown in coastal regions have higher iodine concentrations than those from inland areas. Fortunately the use of iodised table salt ensures adequate amounts of iodine with no apparent risk.

HUNGER AND MALNUTRITION

According to some estimates, half to as much as twothirds of the world's population are poorly nourished. Malnutrition is not just a problem of getting enough to eat. There are a variety of causes, including some you might not have considered. For example, *malnutrition* can come from *overnutrition*. In the United States and elsewhere, many people suffer from diabetes, hypertension, obesity, and other ill effects of rich diets.

Moreover, these people can grow fat from *overindulgence* and still suffer from deficiency diseases because one or more essential nutrients are missing from their meals. The sad fact is that while some people are eating too well and others eating *foolishly*, many more are facing a severe food shortage.

More Mouths than Food

Agricultural production is seriously deficient in many countries of Latin America, Asia, and Africa. And these countries have very little money to buy what surplus food may be available in world markets. Four hundred million people are said to exist on near-starvation diets. Worse yet, according to the World Health Organisation, 12,000 people starve to death every day of the year.

Without doubt, one of the most pressing human problems in the world today is human hunger. It is a predicament of ever-increasing proportions because of spiraling population growth. An astounding million and a half new mouths must be fed each week. And although chronic hunger is debilitating in young and old alike, it is the children that are most harmed by malnutrition.

Suffering Little Children

The causes of infant and childhood malnutrition are complex. Some result from ignorance or ingrained cultural patterns. Others directly reflect food shortages. But whatever the cause, malnutrition in childhood *hampers* normal physical and mental development. Children who are inadequately nourished can be handicapped as adults.

A Poor Start in Life

Immediately after birth a mother's milk meets her child's needs, but within a few months the quantity of milk becomes insufficient, and the child requires substances such as iron that aren't present in milk. In most of the developing countries the supplements provided during the first year or two of life are inadequate.

In many cultures little or no effort is made to prepare foods specifically for the young child. Infants merely receive occasional bits of the adult fare, apparently more to accustom them to the taste than to nourish then. When special foods are provided for babies, they usually consist of gruels of high-carbohydrate and low-protein substances, such as bananas, yams, or sugar cane. Nutritious portions of the adult diet are commonly forbidden to young children in the mistaken belief that they are harmful. Thus the children more often than not receive a nutritionally poor start in life, even when food supplies are adequate. The harm can be dramatic and permanent.

Kwashiorkor: a Belly Full of Empty Calories

Children can get plenty to eat but still be badly nourished. It happens particularly when the diet contains too little protein. Indeed, protein deficiency accompanied by considerable caloric intake is in some ways worse than total starvation. The child may appear plump, though small, but can be seriously ill with *kwashiorkor*. The name derives from the Ghan language and means "the sickness the older child gets when the next child is born." In other words, it is a disease of weaning.

If the diet contains calories but little protein, any amino acids that are available must be used to synthesize the enzymes needed to digest and use the calorie-containing food. This function takes first priority for amino acids; none may be left for building proteins for cell growth. Eventually, there may not even be enough amino acids to supply the digestive system, and the organs degenerate.

Children with kwashiorkor typically have badly bloated bellies, because their tissues become filled with water. The blood of kwashiorkor victims contains so little protein that the circulation is hampered. Fluids stagnate in the tissues, and the body swells.

Empty Stomachs. It is bad enough not to get necessary vitamins and minerals or enough protein, but a diet that is low in calories as well means true starvation. Children with extreme protein-calorie deficiencies are emaciated and dwarfed. The condition is known as *marasmus*. With less severe starvation growth is slow. Poorly fed children are always small for their age.

The effect of childhood nutrition on adult stature and weight can be seen from observations of Japanese-American children. Early Japanese immigrants were small people, much shorter and lighter than Americans of other backgrounds. Over the past three generations the living standards of these people have improved, and so have the growth rates of their children.

Unlike their grandparents, the young JapaneseAmericans of today are not much smaller than other U.S. citizens. Something similar has happened in Japan itself. The postwar years have been prosperous ones for the Japanese. So prosperous, in fact, that the present generation of young people are markedly taller and heavier than their forebears. What were once thought to be genetically determined differences of height and weight were largely reflections of early childhood diet.

With malnutrition comes increased susceptibility to childhood diseases and illnesses. Early death may come, not from starvation itself but from sickness. Sadly, those who survive marasmus are usually mentally dull or even retarded.

Experiments with dogs show that severe amino acid deficiencies in the diet of the pregnant mother or the newborn result in drastic disorders of the nervous system. Because the human brain completes most of its growth by six months after birth, it is little wonder that the absence of adequate building materials early in life results in mental *retardation*. The end result of inadequate nutrition is inadequate bodies and stunted minds.

YOU ARE WHAT YOU EAT

Our food, like ourselves, consists mostly of water, minerals, and organic compounds. Only inorganic compounds are abundant in the physical environment. Organic molecules are rarely found in the world outside cells or cell products. Green plants photosynthesize organic molecules from inorganic raw materials.

They are thus the primary source of organic compounds for most other forms of life. They are the basis of every *food chain*. Humans and other heterotrophs can make organic constituents only when organic raw materials are available. Since cells are the only sources of such organic matter, *heterotrophs* can obtain it only by feeding on others. And because cells contain water and minerals, too, they can supply these inorganic constituents.

Heterotrophs consume plant and animal cells or cell products, break them down, use some parts *outright*, and *rebuild* others into forms suitable for their own existence. You might say that people and other heterotrophs are reconstructionists. Our specifically human nutritional needs are determined by the *metabolic* machinery of our bodies. Human cells lack the enzymes needed to manufacture certain molecules that are necessary to life.

These molecules, in addition to water, minerals, and energy sources, must be present in the food we eat if our cells are to survive. But basically all cells have the same nutritional needs: water and sources of carbon, energy, nitrogen, minerals, and sometimes growth factors such as vitamins.

Not surprisingly, then, most cells-at least, most heterotrophic cells-have a similar metabolism. Glycolysis and respiration occur in yeast cells as well as in muscle cells. The metabolic mill is a crossroad of degradative and synthetic metabolic routes in nearly every organism. And since many aspects of metabolism are widely shared, many enzymes are found in all cells.

Other enzymes are unique, giving cells that have them distinctive metabolic characteristics. Different metabolic capabilities account for the specialisation of cells in different tissues, as well as the differences among organisms.

4

CIRCULATION

As we discussed earlier in this book, every cell in the body of a complex organism builds its own membranes and organelles, makes its own ATP, and assembles its own enzymes and other proteins. To engage in these activities, cells need oxygen and nutrients and must dispose of carbon dioxide and other wastes.

In single-celled organisms and very small multicellular ones, the needs of each cell are supplied directly by the medium in which the organism lives. In larger, more complex animals, these needs are supplied by a transport system. In humans and other vertebrates, gases (oxygen and carbon dioxide), nutrient molecules, hormones, and wastes are transported in the bloodstream.

The blood circulates through a closed circuit of continuous vessels, propelled by the contractions of a specialised muscle, the heart. This system is known as the *cardiovascular system* (from *cardio,* meaning "heart," and *vascular,* meaning "*vessel*"). In this system, the heart pumps the blood into the large arteries, from which it travels to branching, smaller arteries (the *arterioles*) and then into very small vessels, the *capillaries*.

Through the thin walls of the capillaries, nutrients, oxygen, carbon dioxide, and other molecules are exchanged between the blood and the fluids surrounding the body cells (the interstitial fluids). From the capillaries, the blood passes into small veins, the *venules*, then into larger veins, and through them, back to the heart.

Thus the heart, arteries, and veins are, in essence, the means for getting the blood to and from the capillaries, where the actual function of the circulatory system is carried out.

THE BLOOD VESSELS

In humans, the diameter of the opening of the largest artery, the *aorta*, is 2.5 centimeters, that of the smallest capillary only 8 micrometers, and that of the largest vein, the *vena cava*, 3 centimeters. Arteries, veins, and capillaries differ not only in their diameters but also in the structure of their walls.

Of the three types of vessels, the arteries have the thickest, strongest walls, made up of three layers. The inner layer, or endothelium (a type of *epithelial tissue*), forms the lining of the vessels; the middle layer contains smooth muscles and elastic tissues; the outer layer, also elastic, is made of collagen and other supporting tissues.

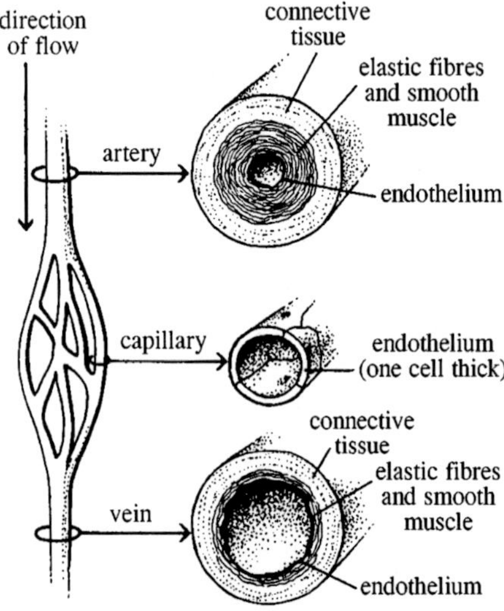

Figure 4.1 : Structure of blood vessels.

Because of their elasticity, the arteries expand when the blood is pumped into them, and then relax slowly; as a consequence, by the time the blood leaves the arteries it is flowing smoothly through the vessels, rather than in spurts, as it does when it leaves the heart. The pulsation felt when the fingertips are placed over an artery close to the body surface-as in the *wrist-represents* the alternating expansion and *recoil* of an *elastic arterial* wall.

Capillaries and Diffusion

The walls of the *capillaries* consist of only one layer of cells, the endothelium, and the *passageway* (*lumen*) of the smallest capillary is about 6 micrometers in diameter, just wide enough for red blood cells to move in single file. The total length of the capillaries in a human adult is more than 80,000 kilometers. Because of the total cross-sectional area, blood moves slowly through the capillary system.

As it moves, gases (oxygen and carbon dioxide), hormones, and other materials are exchanged with the surrounding tissues by diffusion through junctions between the *endothelial cells* and through the cytoplasm of the endothelial cells. Organic molecules, such as glucose, are probably moved by transport systems of the cells. Pinocytotic vesicles have been observed in the capillary *endothelial cells*; they presumably serve to ferry dissolved materials in or out of the capillaries.

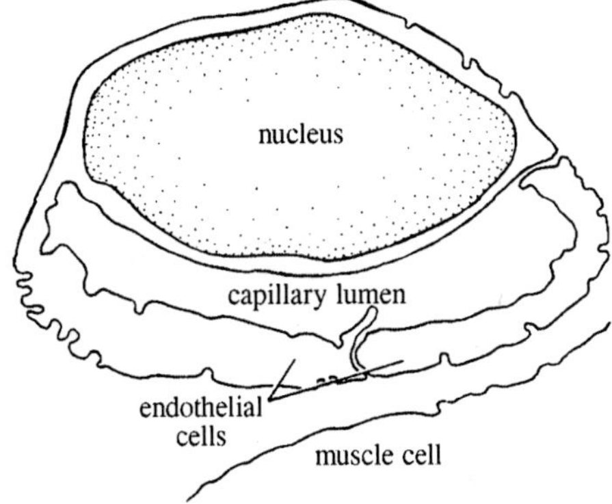

Figure 4.2 : Electron micrograph of a capillary from cardiac muscle. Portions of two endothelial cells can be seen, fitting together to form the capillary lumen.

At the *arteriolar* end of the capillaries, the hydrostatic pressure of the blood is greater than its osmotic pressure, and the watery component of the blood leaves the capillaries along with nutrient molecules and oxygen. By the time the blood reaches the venous end of the capillaries, the *hydrostatic* pressure has dropped to a point where it now is less than the osmotic pressure of the blood, and fluids move back into the capillaries.

As a consequence, there is little total fluid loss from the blood as it moves through the capillaries. (The relatively small amount that is not returned by osmosis is channeled back into the bloodstream by the lymphatic system, as we shall see later in this chapter.) When loss of water into tissues does occur, as, for example, when the endothelium is damaged by a blow, *swelling* (*edema*) is produced. The edema associated with certain forms of malnutrition is also due to the movement of fluids out of the capillaries.

No cell in the human body is farther than 130 micrometers-a distance short enough for rapid diffusion-from a capillary. Even the cells in the walls of the large veins and arteries depend on this capillary system for their blood supply, as does the heart itself, like all the other organs of the body.

At the ends of the capillary beds, blood passes into the venules, smallest of the veins, then into *larger veins*, and finally back into the heart either through the superior (anterior) or inferior (posterior) vena cava. Like those of the arteries, the walls of the veins are three-layered, but they are less elastic and more pliable. An empty vein collapses, whereas an empty artery remains open. The veins, with their thin walls and relatively large diameters, offer little resistance to flow, facilitating the return of the blood to the heart.

Blood Pressure

Blood pressure is the force per unit area with which blood pushes against the walls of the blood vessels. It is conventionally described in terms of how high it can push a column of mercury. For medical purposes, it is usually measured at the artery of the left upper arm.

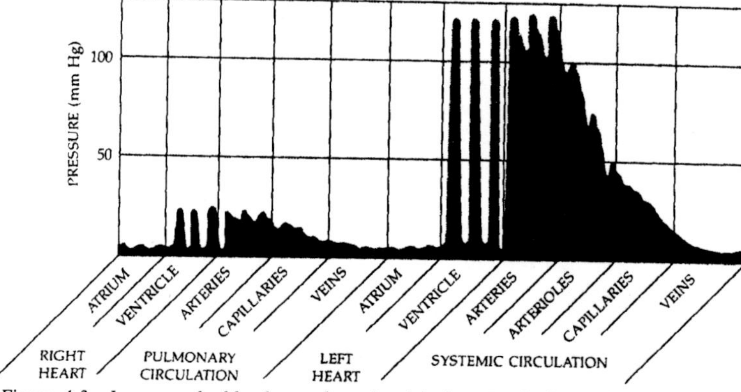

Figure 4.3 : In mammals, blood goes from the right heart to the lungs, from the lungs to the left heart, and, from the left heart, it enters the systemic circulation, moving from arteries to arterioles to capillaries to veins.

Normal blood pressure in a young man is 120 millimeters of mercury (120 mm Hg) when the heart is contracting (the systolic blood pressure) and 80 mm Hg when the heart relaxes (diastolic pressure); this is stated as a blood pressure of 120/80. The blood pressure of a young woman is 4 to 8 mm Hg less.

The pressure is generated by the pumping action of the heart and changes with the rate at which it contracts. Blood flow is directly proportional to blood pressure; the greater the pressure, the greater the flow.

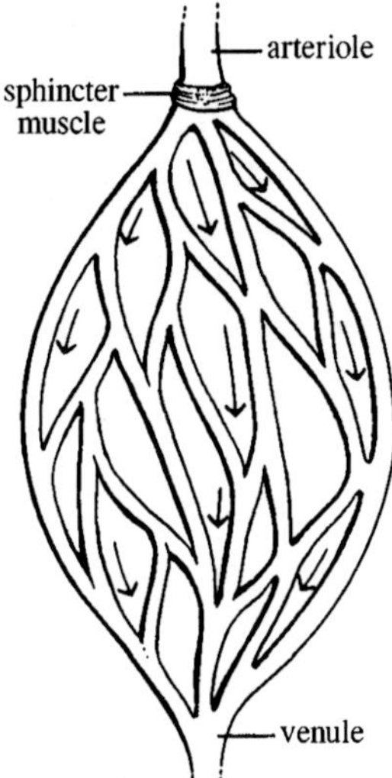

Figure 4.4 : Diagram of a capillary bed. The sphincter muscle at the end of the arteriole controls the blood flow through the capillaries.

Constriction of the arteries by loss of elasticity or by the formation of fatty deposits within their walls increases the *systolic* blood pressure and also increases the work load on the heart.

Blood pressure is not the same in the various parts of the cardiovascular system. As the blood gets farther along the system of vessels, the pressure drops, becoming lower in the veins and lowest in the right *atrium* (upper chamber of the heart).

Thus the blood, moving toward an area of lower pressure, returns toward the heart. Gravity affects blood pressure, decreasing the flow of blood to the brain, as you know if you have experienced *dizziness* on standing suddenly.

Fainting and falling down are protective responses that prevent serious damage to the brain cells as a result of inadequate blood supply. These responses are often thwarted by well- I meaning bystanders anxious to get the affected individual "back on his feet." In fact, holding a fainting person upright can lead to severe shock and even death.

Regulating Blood Flow

Peripheral Resistance

The flow of any fluid is directly proportional to the difference in pressure between the two ends of the tube through which it flows and inversely proportional to the resistance. Resistance is essentially a measure of friction, the friction between the tube wall and the fluid flowing through it. We know from common experience that the narrower a tube, the more resistance it offers to the flow of a given volume of fluid. The exact relationship is given by a simple formula that states that resistance to flow of a given fluid is inversely proportional to the fourth power of the radius (r^4) of the vessel, or flow through the tube is proportional to the fourth power of the radius.

Thus, if you double the radius of a tube, the flow through it increases sixteenfold. Conversely, sixteen times less fluid will flow through a tube of half the radius. As the blood reaches the branching arterioles, the radius of the vessels decreases, resistance increases greatly, and the rate of flow of blood decreases.

Peripheral resistance is the term applied to the resistance that the vessels offer to the flow of blood from the arterial system to the heart. Blood flow through capillary beds is regulated by contraction and relaxation of the arteriolar smooth muscles. These muscles are always in a state of partial contraction, producing what is called arterial tonus, or tone.

These smooth muscles are controlled by autonomic nerves (both *sympathetic* and *parasympathetic*), the adrenal hormones *epinephrine* and *norepinephrine*, and chemicals produced locally in the tissues themselves. *Sympathetic* control tends to close down the blood supply to internal organs and open that to appendages and skeletal muscle, and parasympathetic has the opposite effect.

Thus the oxygen supply can be distributed according to the requirements of different parts of the body at different times, with skeletal muscles getting more during exercise, for example, or the intestinal tract more during digestion. Psychological events also influence vasomotor activities. Familiar examples are *blushing*, *turning pale* with fear, angina pectoris (pain in the chest and left arm caused by a shortage of oxygen to the heart muscle) precipitated by emotion, and erection of the penis or clitoris following erotic stimulation.

THE HEART

Evolution of the Heart

In its simplest form-as in the earthworm-the heart is a muscular contractile part of a circulatory vessel. In the course of vertebrate evolution the heart has undergone some structural adaptations, as shown in Figure elsewhere in this chapter.

Fish have a single heart divided into the *atrium*, which is the receiving area for the blood, and the *ventricle*, which is the pumping area from which the blood is expelled into the vessels. The ventricle of the fish heart pumps blood directly into the capillaries of the gills, where it picks up oxygen and releases carbon dioxide. From the gills, *oxygenated* blood is carried to the tissues.

By this time, however, most of the propulsive force of the heartbeat has been *dissipated* by the resistance of the capillaries in the gills, so that the blood flow through the rest of the tissues (the systemic circulation) is relatively *sluggish*.

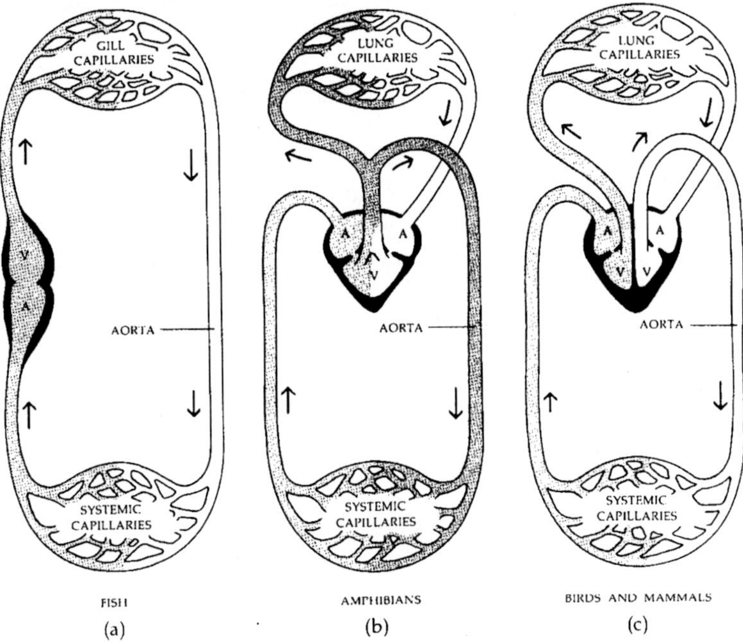

Figure 4.5 : Vertebrate circulatory systems.

In amphibians, there are two atria; one receives oxygenated blood from the lungs and the other receives deoxygenated blood from the systemic circulation. Both atria empty into the single ventricle, which pumps the mixed blood simultaneously through the lungs and the *systemic* circulation. By this arrangement, the blood enters the systemic circulation under high pressure, but not highly oxygenated.

In the birds and mammals, the heart is functionally separated longitudinally into two organs. The right heart receives blood from the tissues and pumps it into the lungs, where it becomes oxygenated. From the lungs it returns to the left heart, from which it is pumped into the body tissues.

This efficient, high-pressure circulation system with its separation of *oxygenated* and *deoxygenated* blood is necessary to maintain the high metabolic rate of both birds and mammals, with their constant body temperature and their generally high level of physical and mental activity.

The Heart and Regulation of its Beat

Figure elsewhere in this chpater shows a diagram of the human heart. Its walls are made up of connective tissue and a specialised muscle-the *cardiac* muscle. Blood returning from the body tissues enters the right atrium through two large veins, the superior and inferior venae cavae. Blood returning from the lungs enters the left *atrium* through the *pulmonary* veins.

The *atria*, which are thin-walled compared with the ventricles, expand as they receive the blood. Both atria then contract simultaneously, assisting the flow of blood through the open valves into the ventricles. Then the ventricles contract simultaneously; the valves between the atria and ventricles are closed by the pressure of the blood in the ventricles. The right ventricle propels the blood into the lungs through the *pulmonary* arteries; the left ventricle propels it into the aorta, from which it travels to the other body tissues.

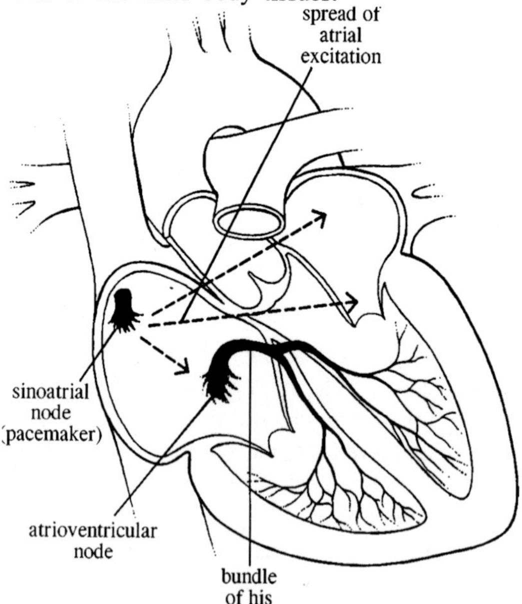

Figure 4.6 : The beat of the mammalian heart is controlled by a region of specialised muscle tissue in the right atrium, the sinoatrial node, which functions as the heart's pacemaker.

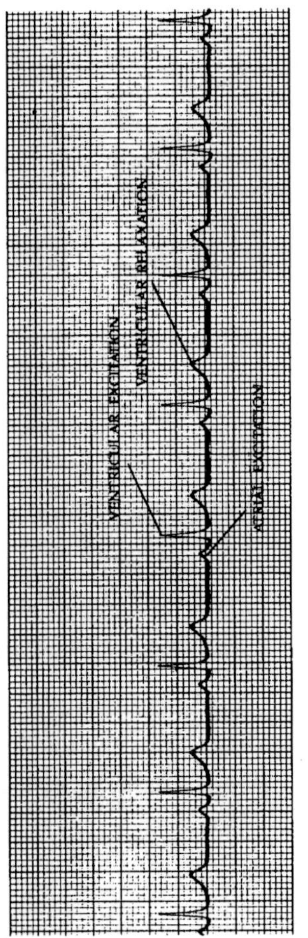

Figure 4.7 : An electrocardiogram showing seven normal heartbeats. Each beat is denoted by a series of waves that record the electrical activity of the heart during contraction.

Valves between the ventricles and the pulmonary artery and the aorta close after the ventricles contract, thus preventing backflow of blood. Most muscle contracts only when stimulated by a motor nerve, but the contractions of cardiac muscle originate in the muscle itself. A vertebrate heart will continue to contract even after it is removed from the body if it is kept in a nutrient, oxygenated solution.

In vertebrate embryos, as we saw, the heart begins to beat very early in development, before the appearance of any nerve supply. In fact, embryonic heart cells isolated in a test tube will beat.

The beat of the cardiac muscle is initiated by a special area of the heart, the *sinoatrial node*, which is located in the right atrium and functions as the pacemaker. It is composed of specialised cardiac muscle cells, which can depolarise spontaneously, initiating their own action potential and contraction. From the pacemaker the action potential spreads throughout the left and right atria.

As it passes along the surface of the individual heart muscle cells, it activates their contractile machinery, and they contract. The action potential travels very quickly, so many cells are activated almost simultaneously. About 100 milliseconds after the *pacemaker* fires, impulses traveling through special conducting fibers stimulate a second area of specialised tissue, the *atrioventricular node*.

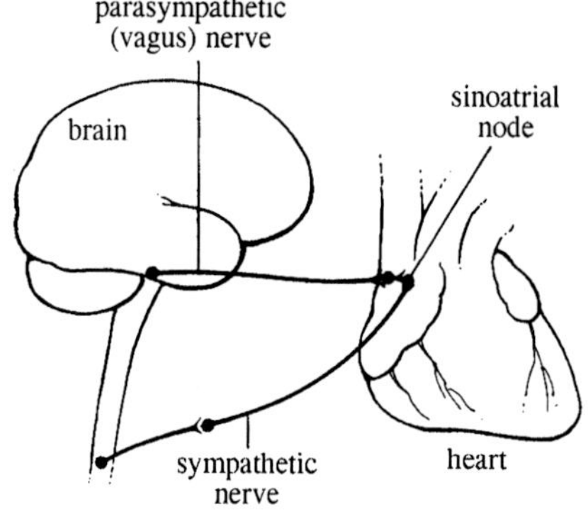

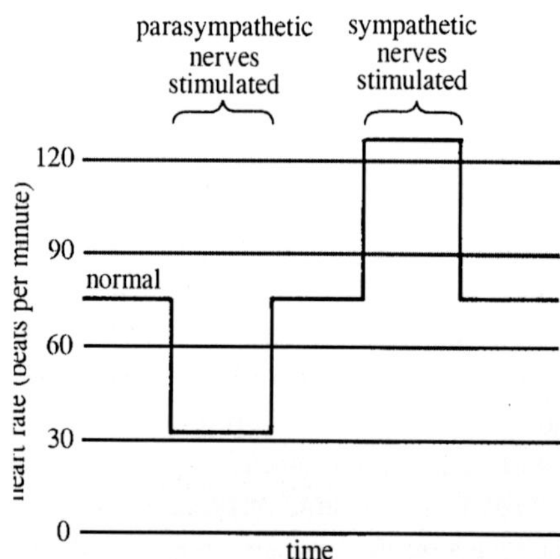

Figure 4.8 : Autonomic regulation of the rate of heartbeat. Sympathetic fibers stimulate the sinoatrial node, whereas parasympathetic fibers, which are contained in the vagus nerve, inhibit it.

The atrioventricular node is the only electrical bridge between the atria and the ventricles. It consists of slow-conducting cardiac muscle cells. Thus the atrioventricular node imposes a delay between the atrial and ventricular contractions, so that the atrial beat is completed before the beat of the ventricles begins.

From the atrioventricular node, impulses are carried by special muscle fibers, the *bundle of His* (named after its discoverer), to the walls of the right and left ventricles, which then contract simultaneously. If you listen to a heartbeat, you hear "lubb-dup, lubb-dup."

The deeper, first sound ("lubb") is the closing of the valves between the atria and the ventricles; the second sound ("dup") is the closing of the valves leading from the ventricles to the arteries. If any one of the four valves is damaged, as from rheumatic fever, blood may leak back through the valve, producing the noise characterised as a "heart murmur" (a "ph-f-f-t" sound).

Cardiac Output

The total volume of blood pumped by the heart depends on the heart rate (beats per minute) and on the amount of blood ejected at each beat, the stroke volume. This total volume is called the cardiac output, which is defined as the amount (usually expressed in liters) of blood pumped per minute: cardiac output (liters per minute) = heart rate (beats per minute) × stroke volume (liters per beat). Thus if the heart beats 72 times per minute and ejects 70 milliliters into the aorta with each beat, the cardiac output is about 5 liters per minute (0.07 liter per beat times 72 beats per minute).

Control of Cardiac Output

Cardiac output is affected by both the endocrine and nervous systems. Epinephrine increases both the rate of heartbeat and the stroke volume of the heart, by increasing the force of contraction of the ventricles. Both sympathetic and parasympathetic nerves act on the sinoatrial (pacemaker) and atrioventricular nodes.

Sympathetic stimulation increases the discharge rate of the pacemaker. Parasympathetic stimulation (by way of the vagus nerve) decreases the discharge rate of the pacemaker and increases the refractory period for conduction along the bundle of His.

Cardiovascular Regulating Center

The sympathetic and parasympathetic nerves to the heart are controlled by the *cardiovascular regulating center*, which is located in the medulla. The cardiovascular regulating center is also the control center for the nerves controlling smooth muscle in the *arterioles*. Thus, if blood flow through a particular body area is increasing owing to dilation of blood vessels, the heart is simultaneously activated to develop greater pressure to support the greater flow.

The cardiovascular regulating center integrates the reflexes that control blood pressure. It receives information about existing blood pressure from specialised stretch receptors in large arteries in the neck (the carotid arteries), the venae cavae, the aorta, and the heart.

The effector organs of the reflex are, as we have indicated, the heart and blood vessels. The blood-pressure reflex is another example of negative-feedback control. When pressure falls, the activity of the heart is increased and the blood vessels are constricted, which raises the pressure again. Conversely, heart activity is decreased and the blood vessels dilated in response to high pressure.

VASCULAR CIRCUITRY

There are two principal circuits of the vascular system: the pulmonary circuit and the systemic circuit. In the pulmonary circuit, blood leaves the right ventricle of the heart through the pulmonary artery. This artery divides into right and left branches, which carry the blood to the right and left lungs, respectively.

Within the lungs, the arteries divide into smaller and smaller vessels that finally become capillaries through which oxygen and carbon dioxide are exchanged. Blood flows from the capillaries into small venules and then into larger and larger veins, finally draining into the four pulmonary veins that carry the blood, now *oxygenated*, to the left atrium of the heart.

The *pulmonary* arteries are the only arteries that carry deoxygenated blood, and the pulmonary veins are the only veins that carry fully oxygenated blood. The systemic circuit is much larger. Many arteries branch off the aorta after it leaves the left ventricle. The first two branches are the right and left *coronary* arteries, which bring oxygenated blood to the heart muscle itself. Another major subdivision of the systemic circulation supplies the brain.

If the circulation of freshly oxygenated blood to the brain is cut off for even five seconds, unconsciousness results; after four to six minutes, brain cells are damaged irreversibly. The hepatic portal system is a special subdivision of the systemic circulation.

Venous blood collected from the digestive organs is shunted via the hepatic portal vein through the liver. There it goes through a second capillary system before it is emptied into the inferior vena cava. (This passage from capillaries to veins to capillaries is called a portal system.) In this way, the products of digestion can be directly processed by the liver. The liver also receives freshly oxygenated blood directly from a major artery, the hepatic artery. There is a large drop in pressure as the blood goes through the capillaries.

The return of blood to the heart through the veins is enhanced by body movements, which squeeze the veins between contracting muscles and force the blood upward. (If you have to stand still for long periods of time, try contracting your leg muscles periodically to move blood back toward the heart and prevent blood pooling.)

Valves in the veins prevent backflow. Also, the pressure in the thoracic cavity is negative (less than *atmospheric pressure*), and as the thorax expands in respiration, the elastic walls of the veins in the thorax dilate, so that blood is both pulled (in the thorax) and pushed (in the veins) back into the heart.

THE BLOOD

An individual weighing 75 kilograms (165 pounds) has about 5 liters of blood. About 60 percent of it is a straw-coloured liquid called *plasma*. The plasma, which is more than 90 percent water, carries a large number of different kinds of ions and molecules. They include fibrinogen, the protein from which clots are formed; nutrients, such as glucose, fats, and amino acids; gases, including CO_2; various ions; *antibodies*, *hormones*, and *enzymes*; and waste materials, such as urea and *uric acid*.

The other 40 percent of the blood is made up of *erythrocytes*, or red blood cells; *leukocytes*, or white blood cells; and *platelets*, which are cytoplasmic fragments of cells. The relative amount of plasma varies among species, among individuals who live under different conditions, and between the sexes. For example, persons living at high altitudes (low oxygen pressure) have relatively less plasma and more red blood cells, and women have fewer red blood cells per milliliter than men.

Erythrocytes

Red blood cells transport oxygen. There are about 5 million of them per cubic millimeter of blood—some 25 trillion (25×10^{12}) in the whole body. In *human beings*, an individual red blood cell has a life span of about 120 to 130 days. New ones are produced in the bone marrow of adults at the rate of about 2 million per second.

Red blood cells are among the most highly specialised of all cells. As a *mammalian* red blood cell matures, it extrudes its nucleus and *mitochondria*, and its other cellular structures dissolve. Almost the entire volume of a mature red blood cell is filled with hemoglobin, about 300 million *molecules* per cell. Anemia is a deficiency either in the number of red blood cells or in total *hemoglobin.*

Leukocytes

There are about 6,000 to 9,000 white blood cells per cubic millimeter of blood-1 or 2 white blood cells for every 1,000 red blood cells. These cells are nearly colourless, are larger than red blood cells, contain no hemoglobin, and have a nucleus. Unlike red blood cells, leukocytes are not confined to the vascular system but can migrate between endothelial cells out into the tissues. They appear spherical in the *bloodstream* but in the tissues become flattened and amoebalike; like *amoebas*, they move by means of *pseudopodia* and many are *phagocytic.*

Table 4.1 : Leukocytes.

Cell Type	*% In Blood*
Polymorphonuclear cells (granulocytes)	
Neutrophils	55-65
Eosinophils	2-3
Basophils	1-2
Mononuclear cells	
Lymphocytes	20-30
Monocytes	4-7

There are several different types of white blood cells, which are classified in a number of different ways according to their appearance under the microscope. Perhaps the simplest method of classification is the one that separates leukocytes into *mononuclear* and *polymorphonuclear* cells. A mononuclear cell has a single rounded or *kidney-shaped* nucleus that fills most of the cell.

A *polymorphonuclear* cell is so called because its nucleus assumes many *(poly)* shapes *(morphe)*. Polymorphonuclear cells are also called granulocytes because of granules present in the cytoplasm. The terms neutrophil, eosinophil, and basophil refer to different staining properties of these granules. Polymorphonuclear cells, like red cells, are produced in bone marrow.

Leukocytes are involved in defending the body against viruses, bacteria, and other foreign *intruders*; they do so in part by *phagocytosis* and also by the production of antibodies. Neutrophils are the chief *phagocytic* cells of the *bloodstream. Monocytes*, which are large cells (three times as large as an *erythrocyte*), migrate out through the capillary walls into the tissues. There they develop into macrophages, large phagocytic cells that colonise the tissues. Lymphocytes are of two main types: B-cells and T-cells. Both arise from cells that originate in the yolk sac and migrate into the fetus.

B-cells, which develop in the fetal liver and spleen, produce antibodies that circulate in blood and lymph. T-cells, which mature in the thymus gland, are involved in tissue-transplant rejections and other immune reactions. In contrast to most other blood cells, lymphocytes have life spans of 10 years or more. Their longevity, as we shall see, is in keeping with their function.

Platelets

Platelets, so called because they look like little plates, are colourless, round or *biconcave* disks smaller than erythrocytes (about 3 micrometers in diameter). They are cytoplasmic fragments of unusually large cells, *megakaryocytes*, found in the bone marrow. Platelets play an important role in the formation of clots.

Blood Clotting

Blood clotting is a complex phenomenon; at least 15 factors involved in the process have been identified. It is not initiated when blood *encounters* air, as was reasonably assumed for a long period of time. The sequence of events begins when platelets encounter a rough surface, such as a torn tissue.

This stimulates the platelets to release substances called *thromboplastins*. (The same effect occurs when platelets touch a glass surface, such as that of a test tube, which is one of the reasons the natural process was so difficult to analyse.) Thromboplastin acts to convert the enzyme prothrombin, a plasma protein produced in the liver, to its active form, thrombin:

$$\text{prothrombin} \xrightarrow{\text{thromboplastin}} \text{thrombin}$$

Several other factors normally present in the bloodstream are also required for this reaction, which involves several enzymatic steps. *Thrombin* converts *fibrinogen*, a soluble plasma protein, to fibrin:

$$\text{fibrinogen} \xrightarrow{\text{thrombin}} \text{fibrin}$$

The *fibrin* molecules clump together, forming an insoluble network that enmeshes red blood cells and platelets to form a clot. The clot contracts, pulling together the edges of the wound. When blood is removed from the body and placed in a test tube, it *congeals* to form a clot. The clot eventually contracts, leaving a clear fluid, the *serum*.

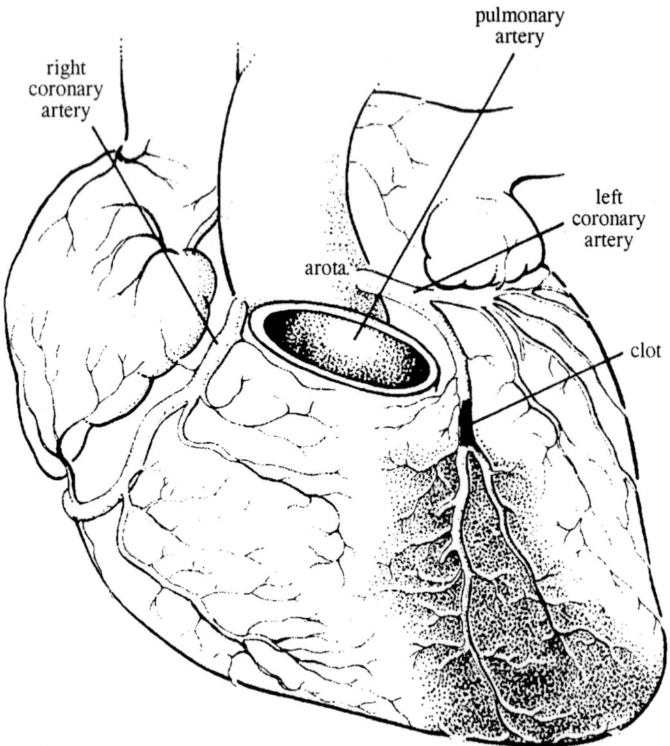

Figure 4.9 : A heart attack. When a clot forms in a blood vessel, the cells in the area supplied by this vessel are deprived of oxygen and die. The severity of the heart attack depends, in part, on the extent of damage to the heart muscle.

Clot formation, although essential to the survival of the organism, also poses a threat because clots can block the circulatory system. A heart attack, for example, can be caused by a clot in a blood vessel supplying heart tissue. The *clot-forming* process is very sensitive; just a few molecules of thromboplastin can set it off.

On the other hand, its many steps provide numerous opportunities for *interrupting* the process. A number of natural inhibitors of clotting are known. For example, heparin, produced by cells of the liver, lungs, intestines, and other tissues, inhibits the conversion of prothrombin to thrombin. Heparin is used medically to limit clot formation after surgery, following a heart attack, or during coronary bypass operations.

Hemophilia is an inherited deficiency in blood clotting. The most common type of hemophilia involves a defective protein (known as Factor VIII) involved in the production of *prothrombin*. *Hemophiliacs*

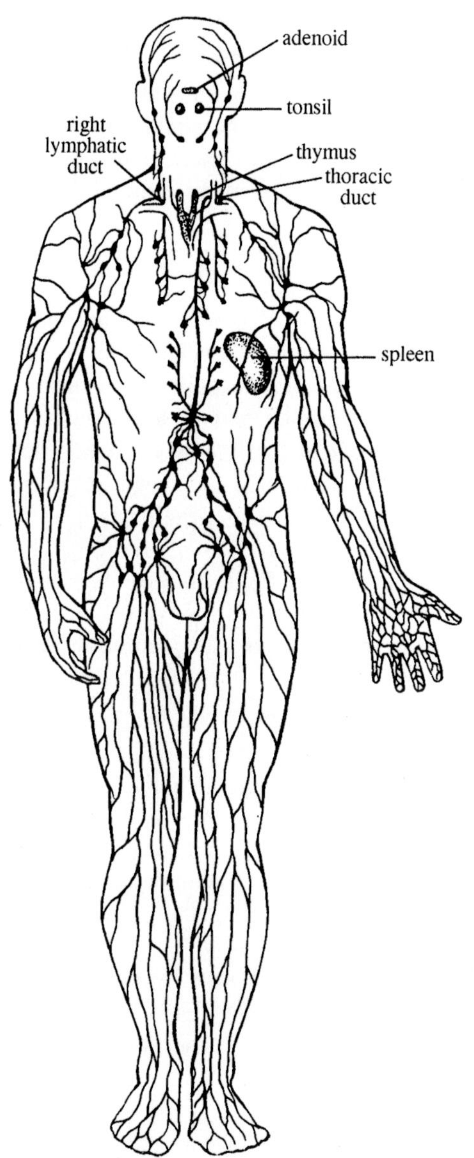

Figure 4.10 : Human lymphatic system. Lymphatic fluid reenters the bloodstream through the thoracic duct and right lymphatic duct.

can be treated by administration of plasma concentrates of Factor VIII from normal blood.

LYMPHATIC SYSTEM

As we noted previously, not quite all of the fluid forced out of the capillaries by the pressure of the circulating blood is returned to the capillaries by *osmosis*. In higher vertebrates, this fluid is collected by the lymphatic system, which routes it back to the bloodstream. The lymph also serves to transport some nutrients, particularly fats, absorbed from the digestive tract and picked up by the lymph capillaries.

The lymphatic system is like the venous system in that it consists of an interconnecting network of progressively larger vessels. The larger vessels are, in fact, similar to veins in their structure. The small vessels are much like the blood capillaries; the most important difference is that, rather than forming part of a continuous circuit, the lymph capillaries end blindly in the tissues.

Interstitial fluid seeps into the lymph capillaries, from which it travels in the form of lymph to large ducts from which it is emptied into the vena cava. Some *nonmammalian vertebrates* have lymph "hearts," which help to move the fluid. In mammals, lymph is moved by contractions of the body muscles with valves preventing backflow, as in the venous system of the blood. Also, recent studies have shown, lymph vessels contract rhythmically; these contractions may be the principal factor propelling the lymph.

Lymph Nodes

As the fluid travels through the lymphatic system, it passes through lymph nodes (sometimes incorrectly referred to as lymph glands). As you can see in Figure elsewhere in this chapter, single lymph nodes are distributed throughout the body, but most are found clustered in particular areas, such as the neck, armpits, and groin. The nodes range from the size of a pea to that of a *lima bean*. A lymph node is a mass of *spongy* tissue separated into compartments by *connective tissue*.

Lymph nodes have two functions: They remove foreign particles from the lymph before it enters the blood, and they are the sites of *proliferation* of *lymphocytes*, which are produced in lymph nodes at a rate of about 10 billion per day.

The removal system is in part mechanical filtration; the nodes catch dead cells and particles that may have entered the body fluids. Lymph nodes near the respiratory system, for example, are often filled with carbon particles from soot or tobacco smoke. The lymph nodes also contain leukocytes that attack bacteria and other invaders. Cancer cells that have broken loose from the principal site of cancer growth are often caught in the lymph nodes, and hence in major cancer operations, surgeons often routinely remove lymph nodes adjacent to the cancer growth.

If *lymphatic vessels* and nodes are damaged by disease or injury or are removed by surgery, fluids that would have been drained off may collect in the tissues, producing the condition known as lymphedema. *Elephantiasis*, which causes severe, often *grotesque*, swelling of the *appendages*, is a form of lymphedema caused by a parasitic worm that infects and blocks lymphatic vessels.

Other Lymphatic Organs

The spleen is largely lymphoid tissue. One of its principal functions is the culling of red blood cells from the circulation. As aged, damaged, and otherwise defective erythrocytes are broken down in the spleen, the iron is removed from the hemoglobin and recycled by the bone marrow for use in the production of new hemoglobin.

In many vertebrates, the spleen also serves as a reservoir of red blood cells that can be squeezed out into the circulation following hemorrhage. Whether the human spleen serves this -same function is a matter of controversy.

The human thymus is a spongy, pinkish-gray, two-lobed organ that lies high in the chest, in front of the aorta and behind the breastbone. It is a relatively large organ in infancy, continues to grow until puberty, and then becomes smaller. The thymus is the source of hormones believed to be involved in the maturation of T-lymphocytes.

Tonsils and adenoids are also lymphoid tissues, which play a role in immunity to microorganisms entering the body through the nose or mouth.

DEFENSE MECHANISMS

The body's first line of defense is its outer wrapping of skin and mucous membranes. The skin with its tough layer of keratin is an effective barrier as long as it is intact. *Mucous* membranes are more fragile, but they are constantly flushed and cleansed with fluids, such as mucus and saliva, that contain *antimicrobial* substances, including lysozyme.

Once a microorganism penetrates this barrier, it encounters a second line of defense, consisting of a variety of agents carried by the circulating blood and lymph. Suppose, for example, you nick your skin.

The injured cells immediately release histamine and other chemicals that lead to the distension of the nearby capillaries, thus increasing their permeability.

Circulating white blood cells make their way through the distended capillary walls, crowding into the site of the injury. They appear to move by *chemotaxis*, the same sort of sensory mechanism that directs bacteria toward food sources.

The *neutrophils*, which are the first to arrive, engulf any foreign invaders by phagocytosis. They literally eat themselves to death. Next on the scene are the lymphocytes. Blood clots begin to form, walling off the injured area. *Pus* may accumulate; it is made up chiefly of white blood cells, dead and alive, combined with tissue *debris*.

The local temperature in the area often rises, creating an environment unfavourable to the multiplication of microorganisms while accelerating the motion of the white blood cells.

Development of Immunity

If this inflammatory response, as it is called, is insufficient, a third defense mechanism comes into play—the immune system. It differs from the other defenses of the body in that it is highly specific, involving recognition of a particular invader and the tailoring of an attack against it.

An organism that has been infected with a particular bacterium or virus is often protected against reinfection by that pathogen. Common examples of diseases that confer immunity, as this phenomenon is called, are measles, mumps, and *chicken pox*. This protection against reinfection is

caused by the formation of globular proteins known as *antibodies* (humoral immunity) and by sensitized lymphocytes (cellular immunity). This phenomenon is known as the *immune response*, and understanding the details of the process is of great biological interest and, of course, of great medical importance.

Like enzymes, antibodies are complex globular proteins. They are highly specific, and their specificity is based on their combining in a very precise way with another molecule. The molecule with which an antibody combines or that a lym

phocyte recognises is known as an *antigen*. Virtually all proteins and some polysaccharides and lipids can act as antigens. A single cell, such as a bacterial cell, may carry a number of antigens, each of which can elicit a specific antibody.

Antibodies act against invaders in one of three ways:

(1) They may coat the foreign particle in such a way that it can be taken up by the phagocytic cells;

(2) they may combine with it in such a way that they interfere with some vital activity-for example, covering the protein coat of a virus at the site where the virus attaches to the cell membrane; or

(3) they may themselves, in combination with another blood component known as *complement*, actually lyse and destroy the foreign cell.

Antibody synthesis begins with an encounter between an antigen and the antigen-specific antibody on the surface of a B-lymphocyte. Following this interaction, the B-cell differentiates into a plasma cell. For some antigens, interaction with B-cells is sufficient to cause the cells to differentiate into plasma cells.

For most antigens, T-cells must also recognise the antigen and cooperate with the B-cells before the B-cells can differentiate. Plasma cells have the capacity to make large amounts of antibody against the particular antigen (and probably against no other). The antigen also stimulates the cell to divide, thereby greatly increasing antibody production.

Division of a plasma cell takes about 10 hours, and the process is repeated nine times in four or five days, at the end of which time antibody production often catches up with multiplication of the infectious organism.

After the first bout of infection, the circulating antibodies disappear, but memory cells sensitized to the particular antigen persist indefinitely in the circulation. Memory cells are primed to begin immediate antibody production against that particular antigen and are responsible for long-term immunity.

The Structure of Antibodies

There are five major classes of antibodies (or immunoglobulins, as they are called by biochemists): IgG, IgM, IgA, IgE, and IgD. The latter two are present only in trace amounts. IgA is found principally in external secretions, such as saliva. IgM is formed early in the immune response and seems to be active in reactions involving complement. IgG is by far the most abundant in serum and is the best understood of the immunoglobulins.

In 1972, Gerald Edelman of Rockefeller University and R. R.

Porter of Oxford were awarded the Nobel Prize for their work on antibody structures. These researchers elucidated the primary structure (the amino acid sequence) of an antibody for the first time.

Each IgG antibody, as their work has shown, consists of four subunits, two "*light*" chains and two "*heavy*" chains. (The heavy chains have more amino acids.) Each of the chains has a region where the sequence of amino acids is apparently common to all IgG antibodies, the constant region, and another, variable region, where the sequence is specific for each particular antibody. The combining sites, it is not surprising to find out, involve the variable regions.

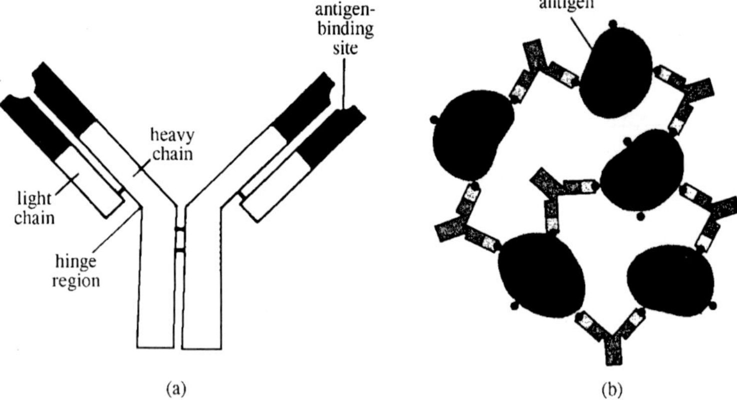

Figure 4.11 : Diagram of antibody molecule. The two heavy chains are connected by two disulfide bridges, and each heavy chain has a flexible hinge region.

Each antibody has at least two such sites, so it can attach to two antigens at the same time. The antigens may be on the same microorganism, or on two different ones. Cross-linking takes place when the two antigens are on two different microorganisms. Each heavy chain contains a flexible hinge region, so the two antigen-binding sites need not be a fixed distance apart.

How do the constant and variable portions of the polypeptide chains become welded into one molecule? Molecular genetic studies in mice using DNA-RNA recombination techniques have shown that in the embryo the C genes (which code for the constant chains) and the V genes (which code for the variable chains) are separate.

However, in the course of development, the genes relocate so that they are adjacent and make one continuous strand of RNA. This is the first discovery that genes can change position on a chromosome and may mark a major advance in the understanding of other events during development and differentiation.

Theories of Antibody Formation

The most intriguing—and bewildering-fact about the immune response is the great number and variety of antigens for which a single individual can make antibodies. An early model of antibody formation proposed that each antigen served as a specific template or mold for the antibody and the imprint of this template persisted, "instructing" the cell in its antibody formation.

This proposal, known as the instructive theory, has foundered as the result of the discoveries that (1) antibodies to different antigens have different amino acid sequences, and (2) the amino acid sequences of a protein and not any external template determine its three-dimensional shape. The most widely accepted theory is that of clonal selection.

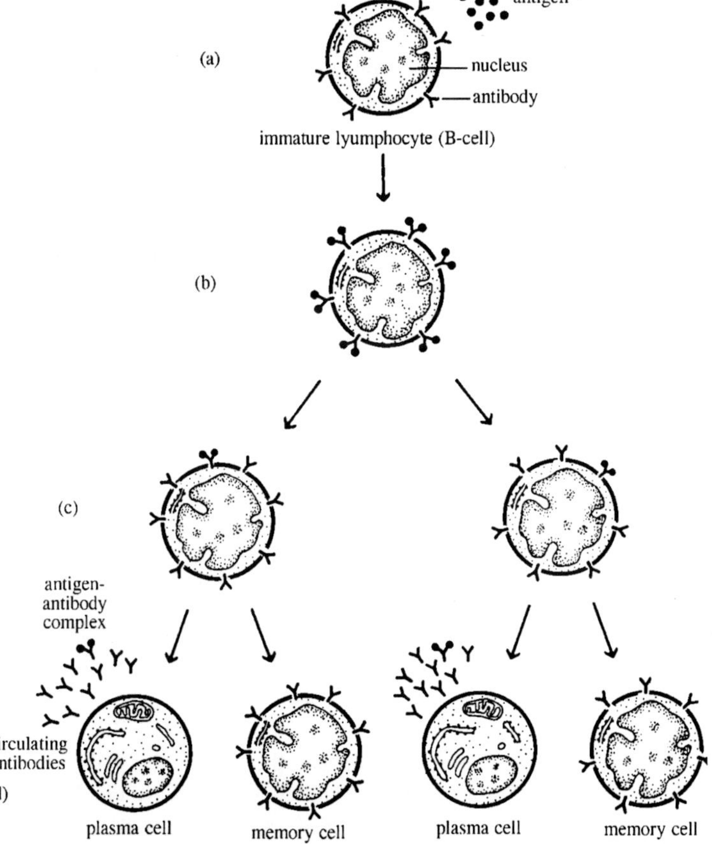

Figure 4.12 : A hypothetical mechanism for the immune response.

According to this concept, large numbers of different cell lines (clones) of lymphocytes exist. Each makes only a single type of antibody specific for a certain antigen. In the absence of antigen, each done exists only in small numbers and makes only small amounts of its particular antibody.

When an antigen is introduced into the organism, it stimulates one specific clone of lymphocytes to multiply and differentiate. This model can be summarised as the one cell-one antibody theory. In terms of genetics, the model postulates that all the genes for making all the antibodies exist in each lymphocyte (indeed, if you follow the argument further, in every cell in the body) and that all but those coding for a single antibody are repressed in each clone of lymphocytes.

This theory has been in some difficulty, as a matter of simple mathematics. A single individual is apparently capable of making antibodies for up to a million (10^6) different antigens.

However, a human cell contains only about 10^4 genes in its entire genome, and many of these code for other proteins. Moreover, the antibody response occurs even when the antigen is a synthetic molecule never before encountered in nature. It is difficult to explain how or why evolution might have provided a specific antibody-producing lymphocyte for an antigen it could hardly have anticipated.

Genetic analyses of lymphocytes indicate that there are only a few genes coding for the constant regions and less than a hundred for the variable ones. Thus, although most investigators still favour the clonal selection hypothesis, pointing out the possibilities of gene combinations, the problem is far from solved.

B-Cells and T-Cells

As we mentioned previously, it is now known that there are two types of lymphocytes involved in immune responses, B-cells and T-cells.

The B-cells are the lymphocytes that mature into plasma cells and make circulating antibodies. The T-cell response is called cellular immunity, since it is characterised by the reaction of the T-lymphocyte directly with the foreign cell or antigen. Cellular immunity to an antigen may conveniently be recognised by carrying out a skin test with the antigen; the skin test used by physicians in detecting tuberculosis is an example.

It has recently been realised that there are many types of T-lymphocytes having different functions. Some T-cells are involved in the rejection of tissue transplants. Other types of T-cells function in the regulation of the immune response. Another class of T-cells (called helper cells) apparently release a chemical that influences the B-cells in their antibody-producing activities. Macrophages (a class of monocytes) play an important role in immunity in addition to their phagocytic function mentioned earlier. They are important in initiating the immune response by presenting antigens to both B- and T-cells in a highly immunogenic form; this is called antigen processing.

Disorders Related to the Immune System

The immune response is a powerful bulwark against disease, but it sometimes goes awry. Hayfever and other allergies are the result of immune responses to pollen, dust, or other substances that are weak antigens to which most people do not react. These weak antigens interact with a special kind of antibody (IgE) that fixes onto mast cells, a type of white blood cell found in body fluids and on mucous membranes.

Another medical problem caused by the immune system is hemolytic anemia of the newborn. During the last month in the uterus, the human baby usually acquires antibodies from its mother. Most of these antibodies are beneficial. An important exception, however, is found in the antibodies formed against a blood factor, the Rh factor (named after the rhesus monkeys in which the research leading to its discovery was carried out).

The Rh factor is a genetically determined substance found on the surface of red blood cells. If a woman who lacks the Rh factor (that is, an Rh-negative woman) has children fathered by a man homozygous for the Rh factor, all the children will be Rh positive; if he is a heterozygote, about half of the children will be Rh positive.

During her first pregnancy carrying an Rh-positive fetus, the mother is likely to produce antibodies against Rh antigens contained in fetal blood that enters her bloodstream. This generally occurs at birth, so the first Rh-positive child normally is not threatened. In subsequent pregnancies, these antibodies may be transferred to the fetus, causing erythroblastosis-a destruction of the red blood cells-which can be fatal, either before or just after birth.

One method of treatment, which is quite an intricate procedure, is to transfuse the infant completely, replacing all its blood with Rh-negative blood so that the maternal antibodies do not cause clumping of the red blood cells. Such transfusions save about 35 percent of the babies who would have died of erythroblastosis. Recently, two medical scientists at Columbia University have developed a substance called RhoGAM, that contains antibodies against the Rh factor. RhoGAM, if injected into an Rh-negative woman at the birth of her first Rh-positive child, destroys the fetal Rh-positive cells that have entered her bloodstream, thus preventing the development of anti-Rh antibodies.

Self and Not Self

The immune system can ordinarily distinguish between "self" and "not self." Substances that are present during embryonic life, when the immune system is developing, will not be antigenic in later life. This recognition occasionally breaks down, however, and the immune system attacks the body.

One type of anemia, myasthenia gravis, and certain other disorders have been identified as autoimmune diseases-that is, diseases in which an individual makes antibodies against his or her own cells. It is possible that other disorders, such as rheumatoid arthritis, the causes of which are not yet known, may prove to have the same basis.

The Immune Response and Tissue Transplant

Because it is programmed to act against foreign materials of all kinds, the immune system works vigorously against tissues-such as skin, kidney, or hearttransplanted from another individual (except an identical twin). The blood transfusion reactions described in other Chapter of this book are examples of this same phenomenon.

Surgeons and medical research workers concerned with extending the use of tissue transplants are seeking ways to suppress or paralyze the immune response in such a way that these foreign but potentially lifesaving tissues can survive. Rejection of transplanted tissue appears to involve T-cells.

These white blood cells can be seen aggregating around a tissue transplant before and during its rejection. X-ray treatment and certain chemicals that inhibit white blood cell production suppress immune reactions. Such treatments, of course, also render the patient more susceptible to disease.

Immunity and Cancer

Cancer cells resemble the host's own cells in many ways. Yet, within the host, they act like foreign organisms, invading and "choking off" or competing with normal tissues. Moreover, they can be shown to have antigens on their cell surfaces that can be distinguished from the antigens of the normal host cells. Does this mean that people can mount an immune response against their own cancers?

A growing number of cancer researchers believe that not only can cancer induce an immune response but also that it usually does so. In fact it usually does so successfully, overwhelming the cancer before it is ever detected by the patient or the physician. The cancers that are discovered represent occasional failures of the immune system. This conclusion suggests that bolstering the patient's immune defense may provide a means for cancer prevention or control.

5

RESPIRATION

Respiration has two meanings in biology. At the biochemical level, "*respiration*" refers to the oxygen-requiring chemical reactions that take place in the mitochondria and are the chief source of energy for the cell. At the level of a whole organism, "respiration" refers to the process of taking in oxygen from the environment and returning carbon dioxide to it. The latter process-which is, of course, essential for the former-is the subject of this chapter. In every organism from an amoeba to an elephant, exchange of gases takes place by diffusion. So we are going to begin this chapter with a discussion of the principles of diffusion as they refer to the movement of gases into and out of liquids.

AIR UNDER PRESSURE

Diffusion, you will recall, is the net movement of particles from a region of higher concentration to a region of lower concentration as a result of their *random motion*. In describing gases, scientists speak of the pressure of a gas rather than its concentration. At sea level, the air around us exerts a pressure on our skin of 1 atmosphere (about 15 pounds per square inch).

This pressure is enough to raise a column of water about 10 meters high or a column of *mercury* 760 millimeters (29.91 inches) in the air. Atmospheric pressure is generally measured in terms of mercury simply because mercury is relatively heavy-so the column will not be inconveniently tall. The total pressure of a mixture of gases, such as air, is the sum of the pressures of the separate gases in the mixture. The pressure of each gas is proportional to its volume.

Oxygen, for instance, makes up about 21 percent by volume of dry

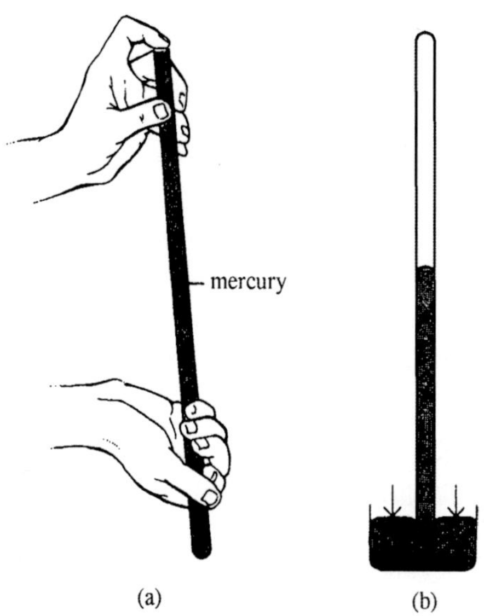

Figure 5.1 : Atmospheric pressure is usually measured by means of a mercury barometer. (a) To make a simple mercury barometer, fill a long glass tube, open at one end only, with mercury. Closing the tube with your finger, (b) invert it into a dish of mercury.

air. Thus the pressure of the oxygen component of dry air is 21 percent of 760, or about 159 millimeters of *mercury*. This is known as the partial pressure of oxygen and is abbreviated Po_2.

In air that contains water *vapor* (also a gas), the volume of O_2 is proportionately less and so the Po_2 is less. If a liquid containing no gases is exposed to air at atmospheric pressure, each of the gases in the air diffuses into the liquid until the partial pressure of each gas in the liquid is equal to the partial pressure of the gas in the air.

When one speaks of the Po_2 of the blood, one means the pressure of dry gas with which the dissolved O_2 is in *equilibrium*. The total amount of gas in the liquid may be very small. For instance, 100 ml of fully aerated sea water at 15°C contain only 0.5 ml of oxygen, or only 0.5 percent by volume.

Thus when we speak of *venous* blood with a Po_2 of 40 mm Hg, we mean that it would be in equilibrium with air in which the partial pressure of oxygen were 40 mm Hg and that, if it were exposed to the usual mixture of air, oxygen would move from the air into the venous blood until the blood Po_2 = 155 mm Hg and equilibrium was reached. *Gases* move from a region of higher partial pressure to a region of lower partial pressure.

Table 5.1 : Composition of Dry Air.

Gas	*% Of Volume*
Oxygen	21
Nitrogen	77
Argon	1
Carbon dioxide	0.03
Other gases*	0.97

We are so accustomed to the pressure of the air around us that we are unaware of its presence or of its effects on us. However, if you visit a place-such as Mexico City-which is at a comparatively high altitude and therefore has a lower atmospheric pressure (and of course, a lower Po_2), you will feel lightheaded at first and will tire easily.

Regular *inhabitants* of such places breathe more deeply, have enlarged hearts that circulate oxygen-carrying blood more rapidly, and have more red blood cells for *oxygen transport*. The consequences of increased gas pressures are seen in deep-sea divers. Early in the history of deep-sea diving, it was found that when divers come up from the bottom too quickly, they get the "*bends*," which are always painful and sometimes fatal.

The bends develop as a result of *breathing compressed* air. High pressures force more nitrogen from the air in the lungs into solution in the blood and tissues. If the body is rapidly decompressed, the gas expands and *nitrogen bubbles* out of the blood, like the carbon dioxide bubbles that appear in a bottle of soda when you first remove the top. The nitrogen bubbles lodge in the *capillaries*, stopping blood flow, or invade *nerves* or other tissues.

EVOLUTION OF RESPIRATORY SYSTEMS

The biochemical means by which organisms obtain energy in the absence of oxygen are not very efficient, as we saw in other Chapter of this book. Before oxygen came to be present in the atmosphere, the only forms of life were one-celled organisms; the only present-day forms that can carry on life processes without oxygen are a few types of bacteria and yeasts.

The *transition* to an atmosphere containing free oxygen was responsible for one of the giant steps in evolution. Oxygen enters and moves within cells by diffusion. Within the cell, it takes part in the oxidation of breakdown products of glucose and other carbon-containing compounds that serve as cellular energy sources. In this process, carbon dioxide is produced, which then diffuses out of the cell along the concentration (*partial pressure*) gradient. This is true of all cells, whether an amoeba, a *Paramecium, a* liver cell, or a brain cell. However, substances can move effectively by diffusion only for very short distances, less than 1 millimeter.

These limits pose no problem for very small animals, in which each cell is quite close to the surface, or for animals in which much of the body mass is not metabolically active-like the "*jelly*" (*mesoglea*) of *jellyfish*. Many eggs and embryos also respire in this simple way, particularly in the early stages of development. However, diffusion cannot possibly meet the needs of large organisms in which cells in the animal's interior may be many centimeters from the air or water serving as the oxygen source.

As organisms increased in size in the course of evolution, there also evolved circulatory and respiratory systems that transport large numbers of gas molecules by bulk flow. (Remember that whereas diffusion is the result of the random movement of individual molecules, bulk flow is the overall movement of molecules in response to pressure or gravity.)

An early stage in the evolution of gas-transport systems is *exemplified* by the earthworm. As is the case with most other kinds of worms, *earthworms* have a network of *capillaries* just one cell layer beneath the surface of their bodies. Oxygen and carbon dioxide diffuse directly through the body surface into and out of the blood as it travels through these capillaries. The blood picks up oxygen by diffusion as it travels near the surface of the animal and releases oxygen by diffusion as it travels past the oxygen-poor cells in the interior of the earthworm's body.

Conversely, blood picks up *carbon dioxide* from the cells and releases CO_2 by diffusion as it travels near the surface of the animal. Thus the gases move into and out of the earthworm by diffusion but are transported within the animal by *bulk flow*. This system is particularly suitable for worms because their tube shape exposes a *proportionately* large surface area. Some worms can adjust their surface area in relation to oxygen supply.

If you have an *aquarium* at home, you may be familiar with tubifex worms, which are frequently sold as fish food. When these worms are placed in water low in oxygen, such as a poorly *aerated aquarium*, they stretch out as much as 10 times their normal length and thus increase the surface area through which oxygen diffusion occurs.

Insects and some other *arthropods*, as we have seen, have evolved a different strategy. Air is piped directly into the tissues by a network of chitin-lined tubules. In large insects, in particular, diffusion is assisted by body movements, which propel the air into and out of the spiracles.

This system is fine for small organisms but is the principal limitation on the size that can be obtained by insects and other tracheal-system breathers. The planet may eventually be taken over by cockroaches or ants, but it is safe to bet they will not be the giant forms of science fiction.

Evolution of the Gill

Gills and lungs are other ways of increasing the *respiratory* surface. Gills are usually *outgrowths*, whereas lungs are ingrowths, or cavities. The respiratory surface of the gill, like that of the *earthworm*, is a layer of cells, one cell thick, exposed to the environment on one side and to *circulatory vessels* on the other.

The layers of gill tissue may be spread out flat, stacked, or convoluted in various ways. The gill of a clam, for instance, is shaped like a steam-heat *radiator* (which is also designed to provide a maximum surface-to-volume ratio). The vertebrate gill is believed to have originated primarily as a feeding device. *Primitive* vertebrates respired mostly through their skin.

They filtered water into their mouths and out of what we now call their gill slits, extracting bits of organic matter from the water as it went through. *(Branchiostoma*—which is believed to resemble closely the *ancestral* vertebrate, feeds in this way.) In the course of time, *numerous* selection pressures, chiefly involved with predation, came into operation. As one consequence, there was a trend toward an increasingly thick skin, even one armored or covered with scales. Such a skin is not, of course, useful for respiratory purposes.

At the same time, related forces were operating to produce animals that were larger and *swifter* and so more efficient at capturing *prey* and *escaping predators*. Such animals also had larger energy requirements-and consequently larger oxygen requirements.

These problems were solved by the "*capture*" of the gill for a new purpose: respiratory exchange. The surface area and blood supply of the epithelium beneath the gill have slowly increased over the millennia. The modern gill is the result of this evolutionary process. In *most fish*, the water (in which oxygen is dissolved) is pumped in at the mouth by oscillations of the bony gill cover and flows out across the gills.

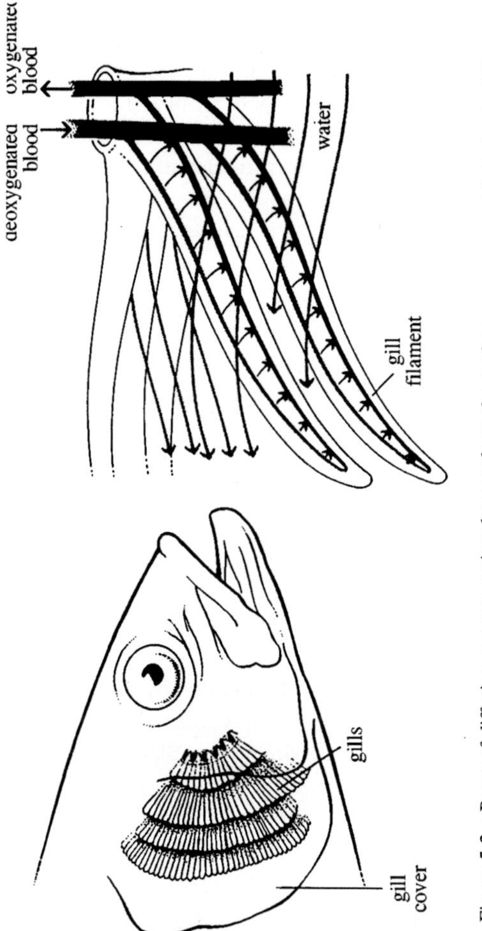

Figure 5.2 : Rates of diffusion are proportional not only to the surface areas exposed but also to differences in concentration of the diffusing molecules. The greater the difference in concentration of a molecule, the more rapid its diffusion.

In the gill of the fish, the circulatory vessels are arranged so that the blood is *pumped* through them in a direction opposite to that of the *oxygen-bearing* water. This counter-current arrangement results in a far more efficient transfer of oxygen to the blood than if the *blood flowed* in the same direction as the water. Also the fish can regulate the rate of *water flow*, and sometimes assist it, by opening and closing its mouth.

Fast *swimmers*, such as mackerel, can obtain enough oxygen only by keeping perpetually on the move. Such fish cannot be kept in an aquarium or any other space where their motion is limited because they will *suffocate*.

Evolution of the Lung

Lungs are internal cavities into which oxygen-containing air is taken. They have certain disadvantages as compared with gills; it is more efficient from the point of view of diffusion to have a continuous flow across the respiratory surface. Air, however, is a far better source of oxygen than is water; one-fifth of the air of the modern atmosphere is free oxygen. Not only must more water be processed to obtain a given amount of oxygen, but water also weighs a great deal more.

A fish spends up to 20 percent of its energy in the muscular work associated with respiration, whereas an air breather expends only 1 or 2 percent of its energy in respiration. Also, oxygen diffuses about 300,000 times more rapidly through air than through water, and so can be *replenished* much more quickly as it is used up by *respiring* organisms. All the higher vertebrates-the birds and the mammals-are air *breathers*, even those that live in the water. Lungs are not essential for air breathing. As we saw, earthworms are air breathers.

The overwhelming advantage of gas exchange across an internal surface, however, is that the respiratory areas can be kept moist without a large loss of water by evaporation. Although lungs are largely a vertebrate "*invention*," they are found in some lower animals. Land-dwelling snails, for example, have independently evolved lungs that are *remarkably* similar to the lungs of some *amphibians*.

Some primitive fish had lungs as well as gills, although the lungs were not efficient enough to serve as more than *accessory structures*. These lungs were probably a special adaptation to life in fresh water, which, unlike *ocean water*, may *stagnate* (become *depleted* of oxygen) because of decay or algal bloom. A few species of *lungfish* still exist, which, by coming to the surface and gulping air into their lungs, can live in water that does not have sufficient oxygen to support other fish life.

Amphibians and reptiles have relatively simple lungs, with small internal surface areas, although their lungs are far larger and more complex than those of the lungfish. The lungs of lungfish developed directly from the pharynx, the *posterior* portion of the mouth cavity, which leads to the digestive tract. In amphibians, reptiles, and other air-breathing vertebrates, we see the evolution of the *windpipe*, or *trachea*, guarded by a valve mechanism, the glottis, and nostrils, which make it possible for the animal to breathe with its mouth closed. Amphibians still rely largely on their skin for gas exchange, but reptiles breathe almost entirely through their lungs.

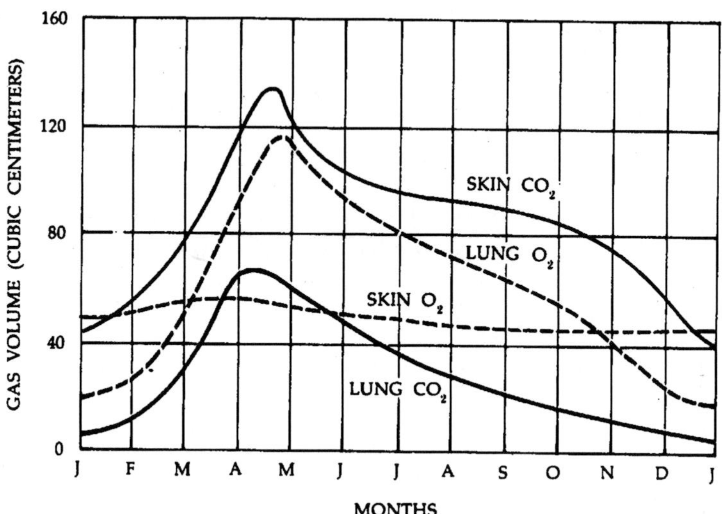

Figure 5.3 : Frogs have relatively small and simple lungs, and a major part of their respiration takes place through the skin. The chart shows the results of a study of a frog in which oxygen and carbon dioxide exchanges through the skin and lungs were measured simultaneously for one year.

An important feature of all vertebrate lungs is that the exchange of air with the atmosphere takes place as a result of changes in lung volume. Such lungs are known as ventilation lungs or air sacs. Frogs gulp air and force it into their lungs in a swallowing motion, thus expanding their lung volume; then they open the glottis and let the air out again. In reptiles, birds, and mammals, air is sucked into the lungs as a consequence of changes in the size of the lung cavity, brought about by activity of the chest muscles. The various types of respiratory systems are summarised in Figure elsewhere in this chapter.

RESPIRATORY PIGMENTS

Blood plasma is an even less efficient carrier of oxygen than sea water; at atmospheric pressure, only about 0.3 ml of oxygen will dissolve per 100 ml of *plasma*. All active animals-and this includes even the earthworm-have in their blood special oxygen-carrying protein molecules, known as respiratory pigments, that raise the *oxygen-transporting* capacity of blood as much as seventyfold. (The only exception is some *Antarctic fishes* that have no respiratory pigments at all.)

Hemoglobin is the carrier found in all vertebrates and in a wide variety of invertebrate species representing many different phyla. A form of hemoglobin (*hemocyanin*), which contains copper rather than

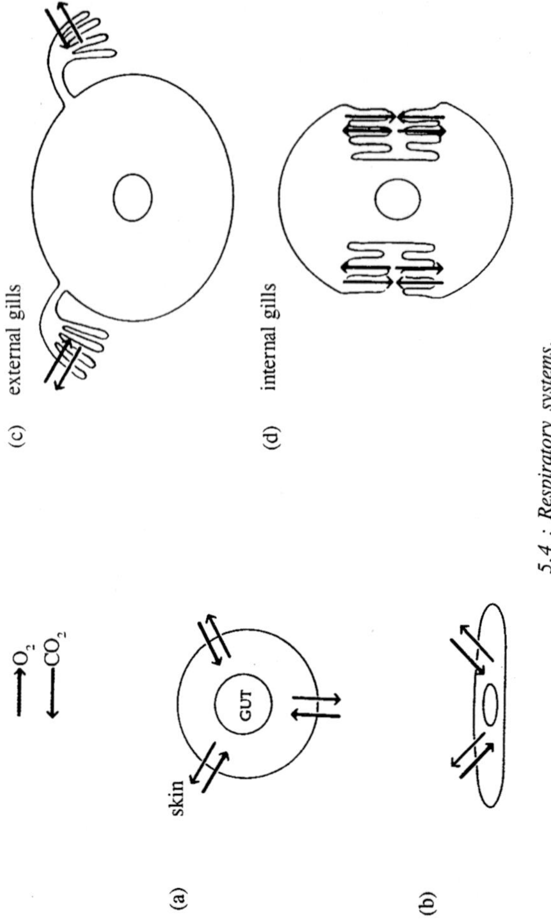

5.4 : Respiratory systems.

iron, is the most common respiratory pigment of *mollusks* and *arthropods*. Unlike hemoglobin, which is red, hemocyanin is blue when combined with oxygen; other respiratory pigments are known, all of which are a combination of a metal and a large protein. In most invertebrates, respiratory pigments are simply dissolved in the blood plasma. In vertebrates and *echinoderms* the pigments are carried in red blood cells.

Hemoglobin, you will recall, is made up of four subunits, each of which comprises a heme unit and a protein chain. The heme unit consists of a *porphyrin* ring and one atom of iron. Each of the four atoms of iron in one hemoglobin molecule can bind reversibly with one molecule of oxygen. The oxygen molecules are added one at a time:

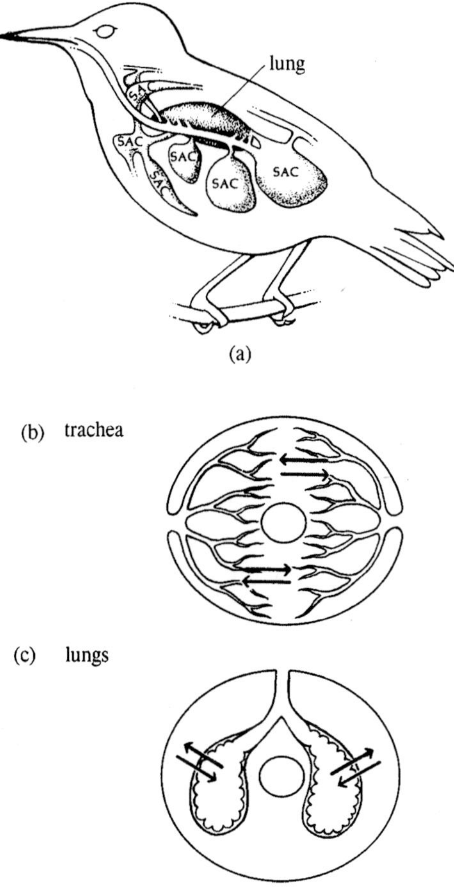

Figure 5.5 : The lungs of birds are extraordinarily efficient. They are small and are expanded and compressed by movements of the body wall. Each lung has several air sacs attached to it, which empty and fill like balloons at each breath. No gas exchange takes place in the sacs.

$$Hb_4 + O_2 \rightleftharpoons Hb_4O_2$$

Combination of the first Hb with O_2 increases the affinity of the second Hb for O_2, and oxygenation of the second increases the affinity of the third and so on. (As O_2 is taken up, the two beta chains move closer together, and this movement is apparently necessary for the shift in affinity to take place.)

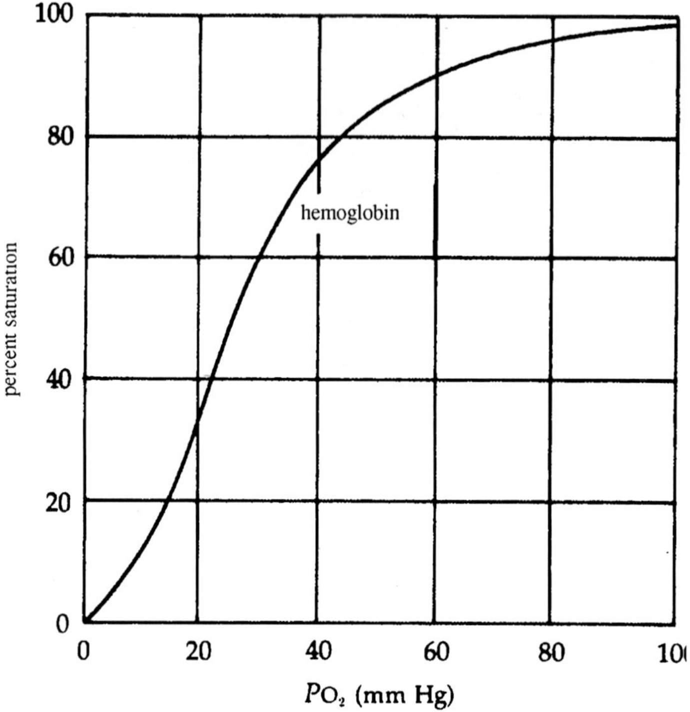

Figure 5.6 : Oxygen-hemoglobin dissociation curve. This curve represents figures for normal adult human hemoglobin at 38° C and at a normal pH. As the partial pressure of oxygen drops, the oxygen and the hemoglobin dissociate.

As a consequence of the change in the hemoglobin molecule, the curve relating the uptake of oxygen to Po_2 is not a straight line, but has a characteristic *sigmoid* shape. When hemoglobin is fully *oxygenated*, the oxygen content of human blood is as high as 20 percent.

HUMAN RESPIRATORY SYSTEM

In *Homo sapiens,* inspiration (breathing in) and *expiration* (breathing out) usually take place through the nose. The nasal cavities are lined with hairs and cilia, both of which trap dust and other foreign particles. The epithelial cells that line the *cavities* secrete mucus, which *humidifies* the air and collects *debris* that can be removed by swallowing, sneezing, or *spitting*. The cavities have a rich blood supply, which keeps their temperature high, warming the air before it reaches the lungs.

From the nasal passages, the air goes to the *pharynx* and from there to the *larynx*, located in the upper front part of the neck. An adult human larynx is shaped somewhat like a triangular box, with its point downward. Across it are stretched the vocal cords, which are two *ligaments* drawn taut across the lumen of the respiratory tract.

Vibrations of these cords, by expired air, cause the sounds made in speech. The vocal cords are influenced by the male hormone. At puberty, the cords in males become longer and thicker, sometimes so rapidly that the adolescent male temporarily loses control over them, occasionally emitting *embarrassing* squeaks. *Laryngitis*, which is simply an *inflammation* of the vocal cords, interferes with their vibration, so you "lose your voice."

From the larynx, inspired air travels through the trachea, which is a long membranous tube, also lined with ciliated, mucus-producing epithelial cells. The walls of the trachea are strengthened by rings of *cartilage* that prevent it from collapsing during inspiration. The *trachea* leads into the *bronchi* (singular, *bronchus*), which subdivide into smaller and smaller passageways, the *bronchioles*.

The bronchi and bronchioles are surrounded by thin layers of smooth muscle. *Epinephrine* causes the bronchioles to dilate; *histamine* causes them to contract. Asthma is a spasm of these muscles resulting in labored breathing.

Cilia along the *trachea*, bronchi, and bronchioles beat continuously, pushing mucus and foreign particles embedded in mucus up toward the pharynx, from which it is generally swallowed. We are usually aware of this production of mucus only when it is increased above normal as a result of an irritation of the membranes.

The actual exchange of gases takes place in small air sacs, the *alveoli*, which are clustered in bunches like grapes around the ends of the smallest *bronchioles*. Each alveolus is about 1 or 2 millimeters in diameter, and each is surrounded by capillaries. The walls of the capillaries and of the alveoli each consist of only a single layer of flattened *epithelial* cells separated from one another only by a thin (basement) membrane; thus the barrier between an alveolus and its capillaries is only about 0.3 millimeter. Gases are exchanged between the air in the alveoli and the blood in the capillaries by diffusion.

A pair of human lungs has about 300 million alveoli, providing a respiratory surface of some 70 square meters, or about 750 square feet-approximately 40 times the surface area of the entire human body.

The lungs are surrounded by a thin membrane and the *thoracic*

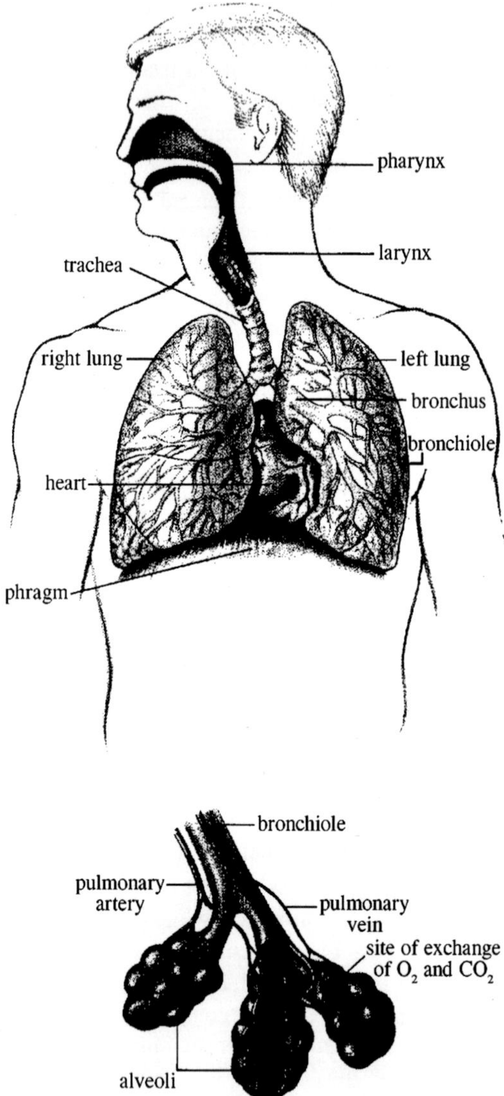

Figure 5.7 : The human respiratory system. (a) Air enters through the nose or mouth and ‘ passes into the pharynx and down the trachea, bronchi, and bronchioles to the alveoli (b) in the lungs. Within each alveolus, of which there are some 300 million in a pair of lungs, oxygen and carbon dioxide diffuse into and out of the bloodstream, through ‘the capillary walls.

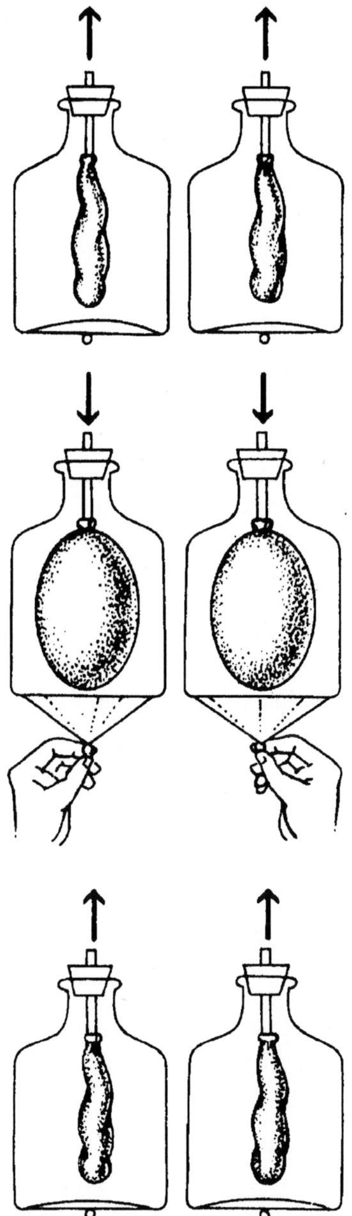

Figure 5.8 : A model illustrating the way air is taken into and expelled from the lungs.

cavity (part of the *coelom*) is lined by a similar membrane. These are known as the *pleura*. These membranes secrete a small amount of fluid that lubricates them so they slide past one another as the lungs expand and contract. Pleurisy is an inflammation of these membranes that causes them to secrete excess fluid that collects in the thoracic cavity.

Mechanics of Respiration

Inspiration and expiration are the results of changes in the volume of the thoracic cavity, brought about by the contraction and relaxation of the muscular *diaphragm* separating the thoracic and abdominal cavities and of the *intercostal* ("betweenthe-ribs") *muscles*. We *inhale* by contracting the dome-shaped diaphragm, which flattens it and increases its diameter, and by contracting the *intercostal* muscles, pulling the rib cage up and out.

These movements enlarge the thoracic cavity, increasing its volume. This lowers the pressure in the cavity so that the pressure becomes less than atmospheric pressure. Air-which is, of course, at atmospheric pressure-enters the lungs. Air leaves the lungs as the muscles relax. Usually, only about 10 percent of the air in the lung cavity is exchanged at every breath, but as much as 80 percent can be exchanged by deliberate deep breathing.

Whales and other large *aquatic* mammals suffocate on land because of the inability of their intercostal muscles to expand their massive chests when compressed under the weight of their bodies.

Gas Exchange

Gases are exchanged during the respiratory process. Oxygen diffuses from the air in the alveoli into the capillaries. As it enters the bloodstream, most of it combines with hemoglobin. The amount of oxygen carried by the hemoglobin molecules is related to the partial pressure of oxygen (Po_2) in the blood.

In adult humans, the partial pressure of oxygen in the blood as it leaves the lungs is about 100 millimeters of mercury (100 mm Hg); at this pressure, the hemoglobin is saturated with oxygen. As the hemoglobin molecules travel through the bloodstream, the Po_2 drops, and as it drops, the oxygen bound to the hemoglobin molecules is given up.

Little oxygen is yielded as the Po_2 drops from 100 mm Hg to 60 mm Hg. This is a built-in safety factor that protects individuals at high altitudes or those who have heart or lung diseases that decrease blood Po_2. However, as the partial pressure drops below 60 mm Hg, oxygen is given up much more readily.

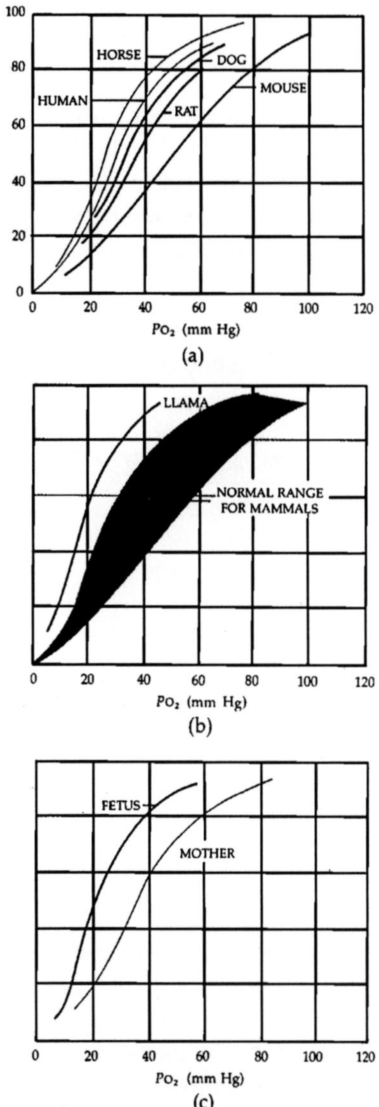

Figure 5.9 : These curves show how the amount of oxygen carried by the hemoglobin is related to oxygen pressure. When oxygen pressure reaches 100 mm Hg-the pressure usually present in the human lung-the hemoglobin becomes totally saturated with oxygen.

The Po_2 of the blood in the tissue capillaries is normally about 40 mm Hg. As a consequence, when the blood leaves the capillaries, its hemoglobin is still usually 70 percent saturated. This extra O_2 represents a reserve supply of oxygen should the demand increase-as a result, for example, of exercise.

Myoglobin and its Function

Myoglobin is a protein molecule with an iron-containing (heme) group; in its structure, it resembles a single unit of the hemoglobin molecule. Myoglobin is found in skeletal muscle. It has a greater affinity for oxygen than hemoglobin does and begins to release significant amounts of oxygen only when the Po_2 falls below 20 mm Hg.

Table 5.2 : Composition of Respiratory Gas at Standard Atmospheric Pressure.

Gas	Inspired Air		Expired Air		Alveolar Air	
	% of Volume	*Partial Pressure (mm of Hg)*	*% of Volume*	*Partial Pressure (mm of Hg)*	*% of Volume*	*Partial Pressure (mm of Hg)*
O_2	20.71	157	14.6	111	13.2	100
CO_2	0.04	0.3	4.0	30	5.3	40
H_2O	1.25	9.5	5.9	45	5.9	45
N_2	78.00	593	75.5	574	75.6	574

Thus, when the muscle is at rest or engaged in only moderate activity, the myoglobin holds on to its oxygen. During *strenuous* exercise, however, when muscle cells are using oxygen rapidly and the partial pressure of oxygen in the muscle cells drops toward zero, myoglobin gives up its oxygen. Thus *myoglobin* provides an additional reserve of oxygen for active muscles.

Carbon Dioxide

A small amount of carbon dioxide is carried in the blood in the form of dissolved CO_2. Some (about 25 percent) is bound to hemoglobin molecules. Carbon dioxide does not combine with the *heme* units of the hemoglobin molecule, as oxygen does, but rather with the amino groups of the hemoglobin molecule.

However, most of the carbon dioxide (about 65 percent) is carried in the blood as bicarbonate. Bicarbonate is produced in a two-stage reaction. First, carbon dioxide combines with water to form carbonic acid. This reaction is catalyzed by the enzyme carbonic *anhydrase* found in red blood cells. *Carbonic acid*, a weak acid, dissociates to yield *bicarbonate* and hydrogen ions:

$$CO_2 + H_2O \xrightleftharpoons{\text{Carbonic anhydrase}} H_2CO_3 \rightleftharpoons HCO_3^- + H^+$$

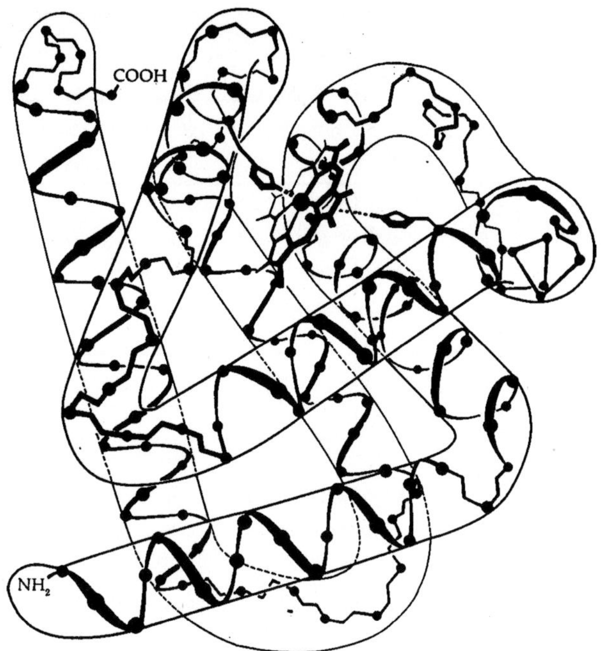

Figure 5.10: Tertiary structure of myoglobin, as deduced from x-ray diffraction analyses. Myoglobin closely resembles a single chain of the four-chain hemoglobin molecule. The heme portion is shown in colour.

As more carbon dioxide is taken up by the blood, the blood becomes increasingly acidic. As the acidity increases, hemoglobin gives up its oxygen more readily. Thus, as carbon dioxide enters the capillaries, the acidity of the blood increases and the yield of oxygen increases.

Control of Respiration

The rate and depth of respiration are controlled by respiratory neurons in the *brainstem*. These neurons, which are in the *medulla*, are responsible for normal breathing, which is *rhythmic* and *involuntary*, like the beating of the heart. Unlike the beating of the heart, however, which few of us can control *voluntarily*, breathing may be brought under voluntary control within certain limits.

The respiratory neurons in the brain become active *spontaneously*. They activate the motor neurons in the *spinal cord* that cause the diaphragm and intercostal muscles to contract. Periodically the respiratory neurons are inhibited to allow expiration. In addition to their own spontaneous activity, the respiratory neurons receive signals from receptors sensitive to carbon dioxide, oxygen, and hydrogen ions as well

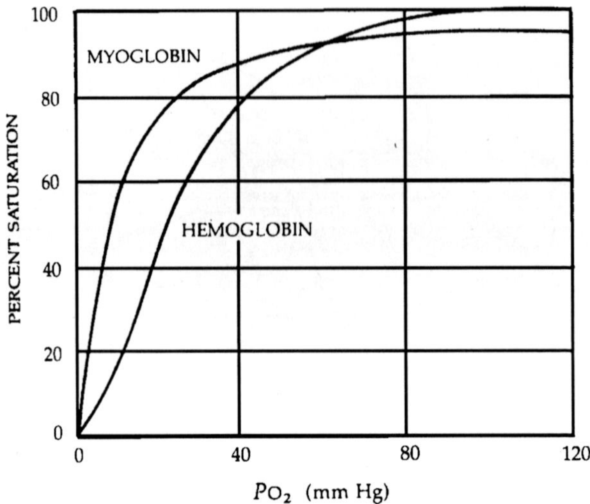

Figure 5.11 : Comparison of the oxygen dissociation curves of myoglobin and hemoglobin. Note that myoglobin remains 80 percent saturated with oxygen until the partial pressure of oxygen falls below 20 mm Hg. Therefore, myoglobin retains its oxygen in the resting cell and relinquishes it only when strenuous muscle activity uses up the available oxygen provided by hemoglobin.

as to the degree of stretch of the lungs. *Chemoreceptor* cells located in the carotid arteries (which supply oxygen to the brain) signal the respiratory neurons when the concentration of oxygen in the blood decreases.

These cells also monitor the concentration of dissolved carbon dioxide (*carbonic acid*), which is simultaneously monitored by centers in the brain. Thus, a number of regulatory mechanisms are at work. Control of Pco_2 is of overriding importance. If the concentration of CO_2 increases only slightly, breathing immediately becomes deeper and faster, permitting more carbon dioxide to leave the blood until the carbon dioxide level has returned to normal.

If you deliberately hyperventilate (breathe deeply and rapidly) for a few moments, you will feel faint and dizzy because of the blood's (and, therefore, the brain's) increased alkalinity. You can, as we noted, deliberately increase your breathing rate by contracting and relaxing your chest muscles, but breathing is normally under involuntary control.

It is impossible to commit suicide by deliberately holding your breath; as soon as you lose consciousness, the involuntary controls take over once more. The receptor cells sensitive to oxygen concentration provide a kind of back-up system for the carbon dioxide sensors. In

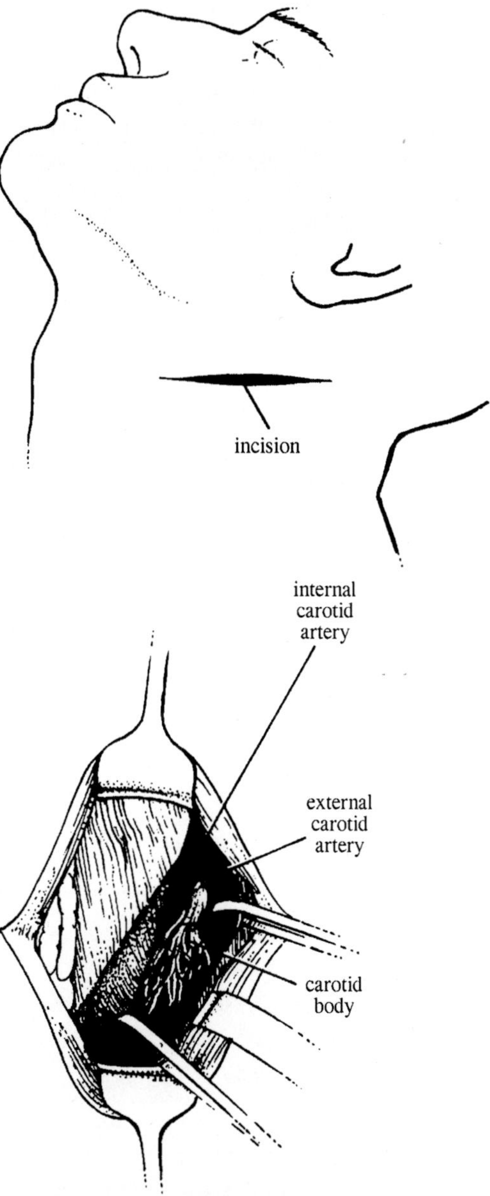

Figure 5.12 : Location of the carotid body, one of the receptors that monitors the concentration of dissolved oxygen (Po_2) in the blood and also, to a lesser extent, monitors Pco_2. Carbon dioxide concentrations are also measured directly by neurons in the brain.

cases of drug poisoning-for example, by *morphine* or *barbiturates*—the brainstem cells sensitive to carbon dioxide become depressed. This causes a decrease in the breathing rate, leading ultimately to a reduction in the oxygen concentration in the blood. The *oxygen sensors* are then stimulated, and they maintain breathing. Massive overdoses of these drugs, however, depress the activity of the oxygen sensors as well.

6

IMMUNE SYSTEM

The earth is really not a very friendly place. You can get yourself killed here. And the dangers are of many stripes, some much more apparent than others. We occasionally hear a story about someone encountering travellers in an alien *spaceship* that has landed on our planet. If such beings did land here, their greatest concern need not be a *trigger-happy* farmer.

Their greatest risks may be of a far subtler sort, such as an *agonizing corrosion* from our oxygen. But in addition to our deadly atmosphere, they might find themselves exposed to innumerable chemical and *microbial* agents, many of which are able to penetrate the bodies of living things and disrupt their delicate internal balances, bringing life to an end.

Table 6.1 : Nonsepcific Defence Responses.

Barriers of the Body Covering:

1. intact skin covered with acids, salts, enzymes
2. ciliated, mucous membranes lining parts of the respiratory tract
3. exocrine gland secretions in surface epithelium
4. acidic fluid in the stomach, basic in the intestine
5. microbes that usually inhabit the skin, gut and vagina
6. lysozyme in sweat, tears, saliva
7. cleansing action of fluids

Inflammatory Response:

1. in damaged or invaded tissues, blood vessels dilate

2. seepage from blood vessels causes local swelling, and also carries with it into the tissues proteins that fight infections
3. phagocytes arrive at affected tissues and engulf invaders
4. clotting mechanisms result in tissue repair

Of course, we live in this deadly sea, and most of us, most of the time, are able to withstand the dangers. After all, we evolved on the planet, and our presence here attests to the fact that natural selection has *endowed* us with certain defenses. Primary among such defenses is our *immune system*, which enables us to resist disease, poisons, and foreign proteins.

There are many immune *mechanisms* in the human body, but these can be divided into two basic lines of defense. The *nonspecific responses* and the *specific responses*. The nonspecific responses are a very general sort of defense that works the same against all invaders. The specific responses are a selective defense, programmed to work against only certain invaders.

THE NONSPECIFIC RESPONSES

In a sense, the skin not only holds you in but keeps others out. So the first line of defense is the body covering. Remember, the basic vertebrate plan is a tube within a tube. The outer tube is covered with skin and the inner tube is essentially lined with a protective *mucous* membrane, both of which are effective defenses against intrusion. The skin is quite an effective barrier, fortified by a tough layer of insoluble keratin.

The skin is covered with fatty acids, salts, and enzymes that present a very inhospitable environment for many bacteria. Other bacteria, though, do quite well on the skin while generally doing us no harm. Their presence, though, means *competition* for any new *bacterial colonisers* that can survive the environment. Furthermore, sweat, tears, and saliva also contain the enzyme *lysozyme* that can rupture the walls of some bactria.

All three of these fluids can wash away potential invaders. The inner body covering of mucous tissue lines the gut, the respiratory tract, and the reproductive tract. The mucous itself entraps invading microorganisms and either sweeps them away by the action of beating cilia or holds them until they can be engulfed by *roaming white blood* cells. In the gut, the highly acidic stomach contents followed by the very basic fluids of the upper intestine kill many forms of *microorganisms* that enter with the food. The vagina also protects itself by promoting the growth of *acid-producing* bacteria. In the urinary tract bacteria find it hard to get a *toehold* for the obvious reason: they are swept away. Although the body's covering presents a *formidable* barrier to invading organisms, they do routinely make their way into our *bloodstream.* (it is disconcerting to learn how many germs can ride in on one splinter.)

Once any organism makes its way into the body's interior, it triggers an *inflammatory response*, marked by a reddening area that becomes warmer and increasingly tender. It begins as the cells at the site of the *infection* immediately begin to secrete *histamine* which dilates tiny arterioles bringing more blood to the injured area. The increased blood flow delivers defensive substances and cells, and *rinses* away *toxic* waste products of the *invading* organism and dead cells.

It also causes the soreness, redness and swelling, encouraging us to pamper the sensitive area until the infection is beaten back. (*Antihistamines* have the opposite effect.) In some situations, the non-specific *immune response* is not localised to a single site, but is systemic. In such a case, the entire body reacts, for example by producing fever. Fever is triggered by either toxins produced by the invading organism or by *pyrogens*, chemicals released by certain white blood cells as they respond to an invasion.

Pyrogens essentially set the body's *thermostat* to a higher level. The increased temperature can make the body inhospitable to many kinds of invading microorganisms. (And so it may not be good to take aspirin, which reduces fever.) Five kinds of blood cells are involved in human responses. Figure elsewher in this chapter shows the major kinds of blood cells and their origins in the body.

Three are phagocytes-eosinophils, *neutrophils* and *monocytes* engulf any invaders in the bloodstream. *Lymphocytes* produce both cells and that interact in both nonspecific and specific responses. The *basophils* secrete histamine that intensifies the inflammatory response. The *eosinophils* primarily respond to allergies and parasitic infections, but here we will concentrate primarily on the *neutrophils* and *monocytes*. The neutrophils are the expendable, *frontline* soldiers.

Hordes of them (perhaps 100 billion) are produced each day and they are the first to arrive at the site of any invasion. They don't survive long, but they may overwhelm an invader by their *sheer* numbers. The monocytes arrive next and once they encounter the invader they begin to undergo remarkable changes, growing and swelling until they become huge *macrophages* (macro, large). These cells are veritable eating machines that may live for years. In spite of their relatively large size, their action is remarkably swift-they can engulf a foreign particle in less than 1/100 second. (The macrophages will also play an important role in the specific responses.)

Interestingly, if they come across a particularly large invader-too large for one cell to handle-several of them may merge, their membranes fusing, until they form a giant macrophage that then proceeds to engulf the invader. The natural *killer* cell (or NK *cell*) is active in the non-specific response. NK cells are formed from large, granular lymphocytes.

They roam the body, constantly checking the body's own cells. When they encounter cancerous cells, or cells harboring viruses, they immediately attack those cells, rupturing their membranes.

SPECIFIC RESPONSES

In the fourteenth century, European cities were *crowded*, *dirty* and *filled* with *travellers*. Conditions were right for a flea-borne pathogen, *Pasteurella*, to sweep repeatedly through the population causing *bubonic* plague, or Black Death. Within a few years, one quarter of the population of Europe had been killed.

A few infected people managed to survive each *onslaught* and it was noticed that, for some reason, they were immune to the disease from that time on. We see the same principle when schoolchildren come down with chickenpox. Once they've had the disease, that's it, they don't catch it again.

We now know they're safe because the immune system has been activated against that disease. Such responses are part of the *specific responses*, when the body is programmed to be *activated* against a specific invader. Two kinds of lymphocytes play a *critical* role in the specific responses. These are the B-cells and the T-cells. Let's briefly set the stage for their roles here.

We will see that the B-cells are specialised to do two things. One type of B-cell makes antibodies to combat the invader. The second type, memory B-cells, forms a residual force that continues in the body long after the invasion is past, ready to mount a rapid attack should that particular invader show up again. (Other kinds of cells, including Helper T-cells, also form memory cells, ensuring a swift and effective response to a second invasion.)

We will also see that the roles of the T-cells are also quite specific. There are three basic kinds of T-cells: helper T-cells, cytotoxic T-cells, and suppressor T-cells. The helper T-cells will interact with other cells to enhance the immune response. The *cytotoxic* T-cells

Table 6.2 : White Blood Cells and Their Functions.

Cell Type	*Function*
Phagocytes	
Neutrophil	Participates in early stages of defense against microorganisms
Monocyte	Arrives at site after neutrophils, transforms into macrophages; Engulfs foreign materials, presents antigens to lymphocytes, stimulates lymphocyte proliferation
Eosinophil	Responds to allergies and parasitic infections
Lymphocytes	
Cytotoxic T-cell	Destroys virus-infected and cancerous cells
Helper T-cell	Stimulates B-cell and Killer T-cell proliferation
Suppressor	Slows down immune response T-cell
B-cell	When activated by foreign molecules, produces plasma and memory cells
Plasma cell	Secretes antibodies
Memory cell	Responds to antigens during secondary response
Natural Killer Cell	Directly destroys virus infected cells and cancerous cells
Basophils	Releases histamine in inflammatory response (as do damaged body cells)

(*cyto*, cell; *toxic*, poison) identify invading cells and rupture their membranes, and the suppressor T-cells help call off the body's defenses.

We will take a closer look at how the B-cells and T-cells work shortly, but first let's consider antibodies and their role in defending the body.

The Antigen-Antibody Response

The cells of the immune system recognise invading organisms and abnormal body cells by certain molecules, called antigens, that they bear on their cell surfaces. *Antigens* are foreign molecules that elicit an immune response in the host organism. When a host is invaded by an antigen-bearing body, it forms antibodies against that antigen.

Antibodies are molecules produced by the host that identify and help destroy antigen-bearing cells. There are several general classes of antibodies. Typically, they are composed of two identical long *heavy chains* and two shorter, identical *light chains*, arranged in the form of

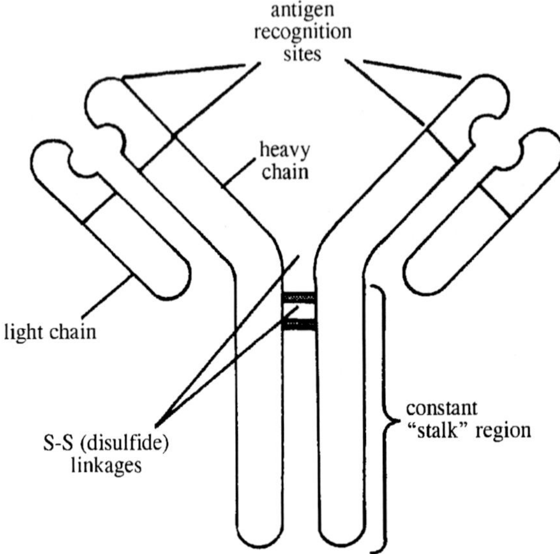

Figure 6.1 : Immunoglobins are proteinaceous antibodies that consist of two light and two heavy polypeptide chains, connected by disulfide linkages. Each chain has two general regions common to a number of antibodies and two highly specific antigen recognition sites that bind only to specific antigens.

a Y. The arms of the Y are highly variable. That is, the molecules of the arms can take any of millions of different configurations (and so it is called the *variable region*). The rest of the molecule can take only a few different forms (and so it is called the *constant region*).

The molecules are placed into their classes according to the configuration of the constant regions. In a sense, the variable region determines whether an antigen is attacked and the constant region determines how any attack is handled.

Basically, antibodies attack antigens in three general ways. First, those with multiple binding sites (with more than one Y, such as IgM) can link groups of antigens together, making the immobile masses easier for the body to deal with (and for *phagocytes* to devour). Second, antibodies may attach to various sites on a single invader, essentially coating it and marking it for attack by phagocytes. Third, antibodies can trigger a set of reactions that *ruptures* the membrane of an invading cell.

Programming the Lymphocytes

Macrophages, we know, are large white blood cells, descended from *monocytes*, that roam the body attacking invaders with a lightning swiftness. But they have another role as well. When they ingest foreign bodies and dismantle them with their powerful *digestive* juices, they take the bits and pieces of the victim-pieces that contain the antigen-and wear them on their own membranes (almost like a headhunter carrying an *enemy skull*).

As they move about the body with the grisly trophies studding their membranes, they encounter multitudes of lymphocytes. Among these are helper T-cells, a few of which have a precise *antigen recognition site* with a configuration that matches the molecular structure of a single antigen, much like the match of a lock and key.

Sooner or later the macrophage encounters a helper T-cell whose "antigen recognition site" precisely matches the antigen embedded in the *macrophage's membrane*. When this happens, the matching antigen and antigen recognition site lock together (chemically, much as enzymes and substrates lock together).

This union *arouses* the helper T-cells to stimulate rapid cell divisions of cytotoxic T-cells and of B-cells that have also recognised and bound to the foreign antigen. The frenzy of cell division in both kinds of cells is triggered by *interleukin* 11, a chemical released by the helper T-cell.

Next we will consider the roles of the *cytotoxic* T-cells and the B-cells, but keep the big picture in mind as we wind our way through a few details: each lymphocyte produced after activation by a helper T-cell bears the antigen recognition site that matches the antigen borne by the macrophage in this way, an army of lymphocytes is formed, all programmed to attach to any invader bearing that particular antigen. This immune defense is summarised in Figure elsewhere in this chpater.

The Role of the Cytotoxic T-Cells

The *cytotoxic* T-cells immediately act against invaders. As soon as they are formed, they begin to roam the body, approaching one cell after another. If the cells are normal and healthy (that is, if they are not cancerous and if they don't carry the targeted antigens) the cytotoxic Tcells goes on its way. But if it encounters cancerous cells or a cell that harbors viruses, the infected cell will be destroyed.

Cytotoxic T-cells then, attack the body's own infected or abnormal cells. As we will see, the next line of defense attacks not the body's own cells, but extracellular viruses, bacteria, and other invaders.

The Roles of the Helper T-Cells and the B-Cells

B-cells have antigen-recognition sites, just as do the T-cells, and so they are able to recognise and attack any particles or invading cells

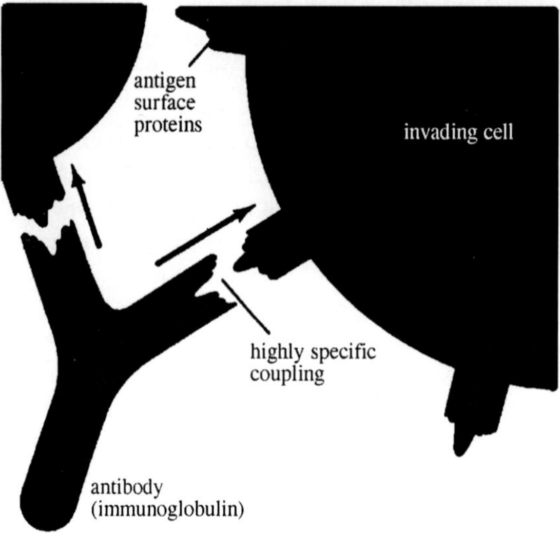

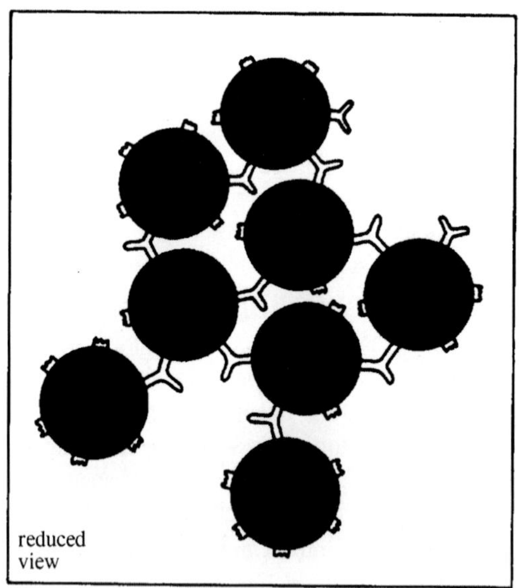

Figure 6.2 : When a specific antigen is encountered, the recognition regions of the antibody molecules attach to specific binding sites on the antigen, eventually forming an immobile mass that can be engulfed by phagocytes. In other cases, the antibody may simply destroy the antigen.

bearing matching antigens. By themselves though, they are only able to hold them, waiting for a little assistance from helper T-cells.

We have already seen that when a helper T-cell encounters a B-cell that has attached to an antigen, the helper T-cell activates this B-cell, causing it to divide rapidly. The B-cell produces two kinds of cells: *plasma cells* and *memory Bcells*.

The plasma cells live only a few days but during that time they constantly produce antibodies against the antigen that their parent B-cell discovered. Memory B-cells live much longer, perhaps for years. If that same antigen should ever invade the body again, the memory B-cells are waiting for them.

The antigen is quickly discovered and the B-cells (with help from the helper T-cells) immediately begin producing new plasma cells and memory B-cells. The memory response is so effective that we catch certain diseases only once. Any later invasion is beaten back before it can get started. As the invasion subsides the defense is called off by the class of lymphocyte called *suppressor T-cells*.

These defenses can be divided into two stages: the *primary response* occurs when a foreign "nonself" substance is encountered for the first time. The sequence that follows the one we have just described (the helper T-cell joining the complex and prompting the proliferation of Bcells that then manufacture antibodies and of cytotoxic T-cells) takes time and so the primary response is a bit slow.

The *secondary response* is the sequence that is triggered by the army of memory cells produced by the primary response. It is, indeed, so swift and powerful that it can stop a second infection before it can get started. Vaccinations often involve the injection of antigens (usually associated with dead, altered, or weakened infectious organisms).

The body is not at risk, but the lymphocyes detect the agent and mount an immune response (often with few symptoms). Memory cells are thus produced against that antigen and so the body is immune to any later invasion by infectious agents bearing that antigen.

Tolerance and Autoimmunity

All the cells of the body bear their own molecular "*markers*" embedded in their membranes. These are different for each person and so, in a sense, each cell bears the individual's genetic signature. As the cells of the immune system roam the body, the body's own cells are identified by these markers and so they are not attacked.

This acceptance by the body's immune cells is called *tolerance*. Such tolerance means that the B- and T-cells do not begin their immune sequences in response to the body's own molecules. By the same token, those very markers act as antigens when one individual's cells are presented to the immune system of another individual. The immune response of the recipient is, in this way, responsible for the rejection of organ *transplants*.

In some cases, unfortunately, the immune system *can* turn against its own body, with disastrous results. When this happens, either T- or B-cells begin to recognise the body's cells as antigens and to form clones that act against them. The reaction is called *autoimmunity* (auto, self).

It is not known what causes *autoimmune* reactions and there may be several causes. As an example, antibodies may cross-react with one's own cells. In such a case, antibodies produced against strep throat can, for some reason, begin to act against heart muscles, causing rheumatic fever. As another example, there is evidence that the body's immune system learns the characteristics of "*self*" at some early embryonic stage.

Tissues that are not presented to the immune system at that time are not learned. The cornea of the eye has no *blood vessels* and so is not presented to the immune system during development. Later in life, though, should the cornea be injured so that its tissue is exposed to the immune system, the *lymphocytes* will be activated and the cornea attacked, causing the eye to become white and *opaque*, often causing *blindness*.

The most common autoimmune disease (affecting about 30 million people) is a form of *arthritis* which is usually manifest as a crippling inflammation of the joints, but can also affect the *spleen*, *heart*, *lungs*, and blood vessels. Autoimmunity can also cause lupus erythematosus (which affects the kidney), pernicious *anemia*, and *thyroiditis*.

Since no one is sure what turns the B- and T-cells against one's self, the most promising avenues of treatment at the present are the removal of the lymphocytes by filtering and the administration of immunosuppressant drugs. (What might be an unfortunate side effect of either of these treatments?)

INTERFERON, AN EXCITING NEW PROMISE

The term interferon comes from "*interference phenomenon*," which refers to a group of antiviral substances manufactured by the cells of most vertebrates in response to viral attack. Interferon causes cells to become resistant to attacks by other viruses. As we saw in other

Chapter, an attacking virus tends to alter a cell's own replicating mechanisms, using' them to make, instead, more viruses that can infect other cells. Interferon helps to block this deadly geometric increase. It does not act against specific viruses, but will inhibit any viral atack.

Interferon from one cell can help other cells to resist viral attack, but *interferon* from one species cannot increase resistance to viruses in another species. When it recently became known that interferon could be manufactured by *recombinant* techniques, hopes in the medical community soared. Interferon seemed to be the answer to everything from cancer to the common cold. But the promises were apparently premature; interferon was simply not the magical cure-all we hoped.

However, research is progressing, and there are promising signs. In one experiment, not one of eleven *volunteers* given interferon in a nasal spray caught cold after being exposed to cold viuses, while in control groups, eight of eleven people exposed and given plain water spray did catch cold. Interferon has also reduced tumor size in a number of patients who did not respond to other treatment.

In one case, two of three separate cancers discovered in one man completely disappeared after treatment with interferon. Interferon does have side effects. In some people, it triggers irregular heartbeats. It may also complicate liver or kidney problems. In high doses, interferon can cause mental confusion, change brain waves, and can bring on seizures. Nonetheless, it is still considered a potentially useful substance and may become a superb form of treatment for some ills, when we learn more about it.

AIDS: A DEVASTATING NEW PROBLEM

Not long ago, an accused murderer was led into a courtroom by a sheriff's deputy who was wearing rubber gloves. The *jurors* facing the *accused* did not include the fourteen people who had asked to be excused because of the medical conditions of the accused. The unusual circumstances arose because the defendant was guilty of having AIDS.

The "*rubber gloves treatment*" is disconcertingly routine in other areas, even those in which AIDS is extremely unlikely. The fear of AIDS now probably surpasses the fear of flying. Sexual behaviour in the United States has changed, it has been said, not by messages from the pulpits so much as by messages from the Centers for Disease Control.

Not only is casual sex avoided by most informed people, but people with AIDS or those in high risk groups, are often shunned, even by those in the health services community. The argument regarding the *contagion* of the virus seems to be more *vigorous* outside the medical community, however, because most researchers in the area seem to agree that the virus is not particularly contagious if certain simple *safeguards* are taken. But what is AIDS? What is the problem? And what are the safeguards? And if it's not so contagious, why are so many people dying?

AIDS is an acronym for acquired *Immune deficiency syndrome*. Essentially, it acts by suppressing the victim's immune system. People with AIDS are susceptible to virtually any disease in fact, the appearance of rare diseases such as Kaposi's *sarcoma* (a skin cancer) and *pneumocystic pneumonia* frequently occur with the virus. Early signs of AIDS include a series of lingering, simple colds, "*night sweats*," persistent fever, *swollen glands*, and coughing. (Immediately upon learning this, of course, everyone detects just those symptoms in themselves.)

More serious conditions follow, including at least three forms of cancer and destruction of the lungs and brain. By some accounts, the first case of AIDS in the United States appeared in 1979, followed by a half-dozen cases reported in Los Angeles in 1981. In early 1989, the World Health Organisation estimated that over one new case of AIDS was developing each minute, worldwide, with 1 million new cases of AIDS expected to be reported by 1993. (The figures have since been revised upward.)

It is estimated that between 6 and 10 million people are presently affected with the virus but do not yet show symptoms (which may not appear for years after infection). Many people carry antibodies to AIDS, showing that they have been exposed to it, and some may carry the virus in its early stages without developing the symptoms. It is feared that such people may be able to transmit the *syndrome*, nonetheless.

Furthermore, one quarter of a group of high risk men who had tested negative for the antibody, were found to be carrying the virus. The syndrome, once full-blown, is believed to be incurable and to virtually always cause death within a few years (fewer than fourteen percent of victims survive past three years). Because so much is unknown about AIDS, much of what is known is misconstrued, often by sensationalist media. Who, then, is at risk, and how does the syndrome progress?

AIDS is largely confined to homosexual men and intravenous drug abusers. The agent, a virus, is transmitted in the blood and semen, but is also found in *sweat*, *tears* and *mucus*. The primary means of *contagion* is believed to be anal *intercourse*, when the delicate tissues of the bowel are likely to be *injured*, allowing the virus to enter the blood through broken vessels. *Vaginal* intercourse with an infected man is less risky for the woman because the vaginal wall is normally not abraded during the act. *Heterosexual* men are normally not at great risk because, at least in the United States, relatively few women *harbor* the virus and *normal sexual* intercourse does not usually involve access to the man's *bloodstream*.

The drug abusers may pass the virus along by sharing infected needles. One problem here is that those in the drug subculture are among the least informed people in our society and so they often continue their practices out of *sheer ignorance*. Some *addicts* have taken to dipping their needles in bleach before each use, but even this precaution is not entirely effective. Others are infected by the "*batch*" itself. That is, by injecting contaminated drugs.

There have been cases of people contracting AIDS through medical blood *transfusions*, but careful screening and processing of blood is reducing this risk. The risk of contracting the virus through *heterosexual* vaginal intercourse is extremely low but on the rise. One problem is the dependence on *condoms* as a protection.

Some types of condoms are not effective. For example, those made of animal membranes, rather than rubber, do not block the passage of viruses. Also, unfortunately, some men simply do not know how to use them safely. (They must be removed from the vagina immediately after *ejaculation*.) There are also other means of entrance to the heterosexual population. Some women have even been infected by artifical *inseminat-ion*. And, sadly, AIDS can be contracted by the fetus while still in the uterus.

The geographical source of AIDS is not entirely established, but some researchers believe the virus is a mutant of a strain that infects the African *green monkey*, a species that lives in close contact with humans in West Africa. The condition is widespread in certain areas there. Certain *Frenchspeaking* and AIDS-ridden nations of West Africa have developed exchange programs with Haiti, a favourite vacation area of American homosexuals, and AIDS may have spread to America in this way.

One problem with tracing the movement, sources, and modes of transmission of the virus is that people tend to be less than honest about their sexual behaviour. For example, almost all the hundred or so AIDS victims in the American military claim to have contracted the disease from prostitutes. Of course to say otherwise would be grounds for *prosecution* and discharge. At present, the American Centers for Disease Control maintain that AIDS is not likely to sweep through the general population, but is likely to continue to be transmitted through its present means.

In West Africa, the condition affects men and women in roughly equal numbers, but it has been pointed out that heterosexual anal intercourse is common there (often after ritual *clitorectomy*).

The problem of AIDS all too clearly illustrates the challenges presented to our immune systems. Not only must our own bodies fend off the usual agents that have attacked our delicate systems over *evolutionary* time, but they must stand ready to meet the new challenges that can be expected in the changing world of living things.

MIND AND BODY

We've discussed the immune system here in very mechanical terms (A triggers B which with C causes D). It's all very tidy, even when we point out those areas that we don't really understand. It appears, though, that if we are to even truly understand the immune system, we're going to have to come to *grips* with how it is affected by the mind.

The very consideration of this topic is met with great resistance in some *scientific circles*, largely because of the "pop psychology" atmosphere that often surrounds such musings. We hear things like "You're as young as you think you are"-this often to octogenarians. (Or, "He thinks he's dead and I hope he's right because we buried him"). Nonetheless, serious researchers are giving increasing credence to the notion that our physical well-being and, in particular, our immune system, is influenced by our state of mind.

People have long noticed a relationship between mood and illness. *Depressed* people seem to get sick more often than happy, cheerful people. Bereaved people also tend to be ill more often than others do. In a study designed to test this relationship, a group of men were tested, all of whom had wives dying of breast cancer.

One month after the death of the wife, the husbands' white blood cell count dropped drastically and with their immune systems thereby depressed, the men began to fall ill. The WBC count generally return to normal after about a year. Elderly people who had been forced to relocate also showed a reduction in their white blood cells for a time. Even astronauts (the picture of health) after being subjected to the stress of manned flight, showed lower WBC counts.

The link between the mind and the immune system has even been shown in other species. In an experiment, mice were fed *chocolate* milk and then *injected* with an immune system suppressor. After several such experiments, the mice would get sick from infection at the scent of chocolate milk, their immune systems in *disarray*.

The link between the mind and the body's immunity was building in the minds of some scientists. With evidence of such a link, the next step would be to control one's mind in order to stay healthy, and many *people* are attempting to do just that. As an example, the recurrence of *herpes* has been linked to the mind. Episodes are often *triggered* by either emotional or physical stress.

Some sufferers, though, report that by relaxation, humor and optimism (perhaps induced *hypnotically*) they can thwart the onset of the *episodes* even after the first *symptoms* have appeared. The mental set most conducive to good health seems to be a positive, *optimistic* attitude. Author Norman Cousins, who claimed to have beat heart disease with, among other things, music and Woody Allen videos, subscribes to what he calls a "joyous belief in an outcome".

But how could mind influence immunity? What could the mechanism be? The answer isn't clear yet, but scientists have discovered that *neuropeptides*, once believed to be restricted to the brain, are found throughout the body. Furthermore, they are chemically related to substances that help regulate the immune system. Some researchers suggest that neuropeptides are the link between the immune system and the brain.

Most of us wish to live long and well. But that implies a continuing existence on an essentially *hostile* planet. Furthermore, that hostility may be increasing, largely because of our own behaviour. Not only are our increasing numbers on the planet threatening our individual access to resources that contribute to good health, but each additional person might be considered a potential reservoir for some mutant threat.

Crowding, of course, goes hand-in-hand with contagion, and we grow more crowded daily. In addition, we must rely on new technologies to help us solve our immediate problems, and the earth is becoming *permeated* with technology's by-products.

We are forced to stand against a tide of chemical agents that are totally new to the environment, and that tide rises daily. Indeed, our immune systems, our ability to withstand, may soon be tested in ways we can only imagine.

7

NERVOUS SYSTEM

Humans almost seem to worship *intelligence* and that great, gray orb from which it stems-the brain. However, a certain irony arises here because we don't even know what intelligence is. People have been wrestling for years to define it and measure it. The result has been sharp *disagreement* and a complete lack of consensus. And when we try to broach the idea of intelligence in other species, the conversation becomes a shambles.

Yet we believe that intelligence, whatever it is, is good-at least for us. And we believe that it somehow resides in the brain. In our consideration of the brain and other neural structures, we will first review various types of nervous systems, from simple to complex.

We could say from "*lower*" to "*higher*," except that the terms lead to unfortunate misunderstandings. "Higher," in the minds of many people, implies any characteristic similar to those of humans, such as a large "thinking" center.

The implication of this usage is that all species tend To evolve toward humallike characteristics, including higher intelligence. Nothing could be further from the truth.

THE EVOLUTION OF NERVOUS SYSTEMS

Clues to the evolutionary development of nervous systems can be gleaned from a cross-species survey from simple to complex. One of the simplest nervous systems is that of *cnidarians* such as the fresh-water *Hydra*. It consists simply of a two-dimensional net of intercon-necting *neurons*, or *nerve cells*, spread throughout the outer body layer.

The entire surface of the animal is about equally covered. There is no part that controls the rest; no nerve center that functions in the regulation or coordination of the nerve net. Thus, if one part of the animal is stim-ulated, the entire body responds and shows awareness of the stimulus.

The flatworm has a somewhat more specialized nervous system. The neurons are arranged in two longitudinal nerves connected by *transverse nerves*, producing a "*ladder*" as opposed to the Hydra's "net." Your keen eye will undoubtedly also have noted the aggregation of nerves in the head region.

These are the *cephalic* (head) *ganglia*, which are composed of clumps of neural cell bodies. As these become relatively larger and more complex in other species, they eventually are referred to as the brain. As a brief aside, you may have wondered why the brain is located in the head. There have been *exceptions*, such as the huge, *herbivorous*

Table 7.1 : Parts of the Nervous System.

Central Nervous System	
Brain	Integration; association; thought, directs most behaviour
Spinal Cord	Carries messages to and from brain; center for spinal reflexes
Peripheral Nervous System	
Somatic Nervous System	Primarily involved in sensations and actions of which we are conscious
cranial nerves	Service the head region
spinal nerves	Service the body region
dorsal nerve root	Houses sensory neurons
ventral nerve root	Houses motor neurons
Autonomic Nervous System	Controls involuntary activities of internal organs
sympathetic nervous system	Fight or flight reactions
parasympathetic nervous system	Returns the body to ''normal state after emergency, controls activity of organs under nonstressful conditions

dinosaur, the *Brontosaurus*, which had a second "*brain*" at the base of its tail to help direct its immense body as it browsed in *prehistoric* lakes. But the evolutionary reason for nerve centers in the anterior, or head, region may have been to permit quick analysis of the environment

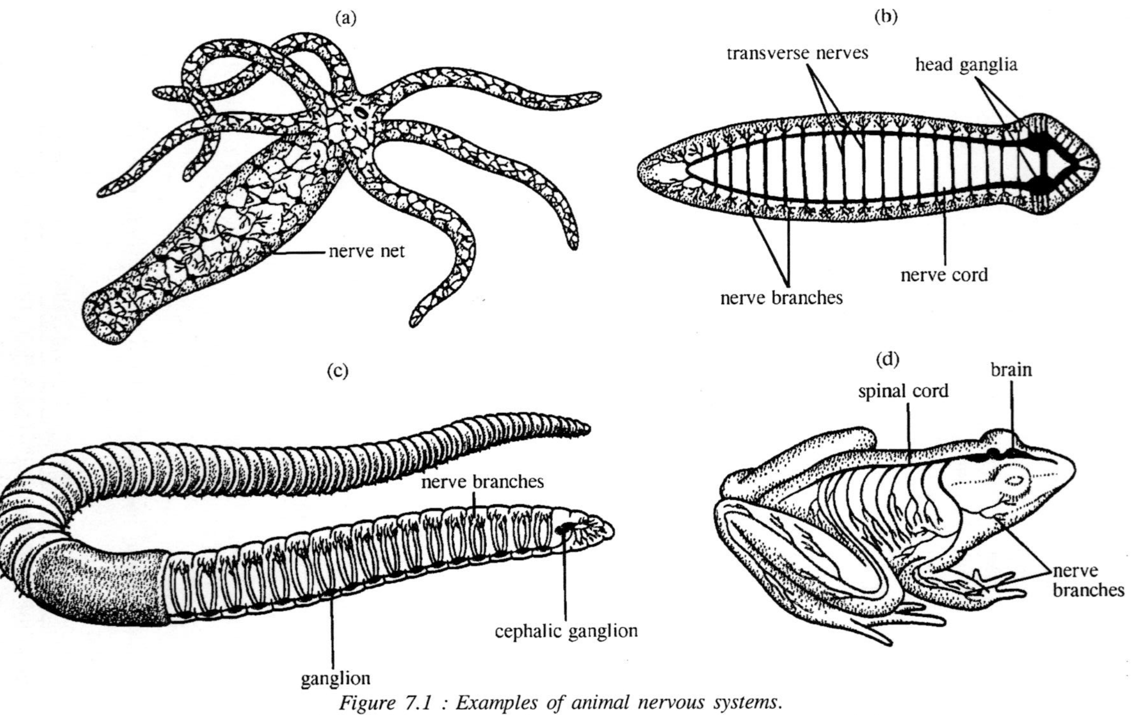

Figure 7.1 : Examples of animal nervous systems.
It is likely that the evolutionary route of vertebrate nervous systems was much the same.

into which the animal would be moving. These centers would in all probability have come to be associated with the *specialised* receptors we refer to as the senses. And as we know, the senses of sight, sound, smell, and hearing are commonly located in the head region.

Thus, the environment into which the animal is moving may be quickly assessed. If the brain and these special receptors were located at the posterior end, the animal might find itself in an *inhospitable* environment by the time it realised its *predicament*. A somewhat more complex *nervous system* is found in the earthworm.

The *earthworm* has a single longitudinal nerve, but it shows vestiges of a paired arrangement in that it is *two-lobed*, much like two cords pressed together. The nerve is ventral, with the heart and digestive tract lying dorsal to it. Note the *distinctness* of the cerebral ganglia and the obvious nodes along the nerve cord, each with paired nerves reaching into a segment of the body.

The frog nervous system is relatively primitive for that of a vertebrate, but it can be used to illustrate the basic neural plan in vertebrates. In this group, we find a distinct brain and *spinal cord*.

THE CENTRAL NERVOUS SYSTEM

The brain and spinal cord together form the *central nervous system*. In all vertebrates, the *longitudinal* nerve (the spinal cord) is dorsal, hollow, filled with fluid, and protected by bone. The anterior end is marked by a brain, an *elaboration* of the primitive *ganglionic* mass of ancient forebears.

The vertebrate brain shows marked *specialisation*; that is, different parts of it are associated with very specific functions. The central nervous system of *vertebrates* shows traces of the paired and segmented neural arrangements of their distant ancestors. For example, the brain is *twolobed* and paired nerves extend from it and from the spinal cord.

However, the paired branching is no longer so regular and apparent because of specialisation along the spinal cord as the vertebrate body plan became more complex. Table elsewhere in this chapter summarises the different nervous systems of the human body.

The Spinal Cord and the Reflex Arc

If you pride yourself on being a "*thinking animal*," you may be a little *disappointed* to realise that your spinal cord can often receive information from the body's receptors, process it, and initiate the proper response before your brain even "*knows*" what has happened. The neural connections that permit this are called a *reflex arc. Physicians* often like to tap the tendon below the knee, making the leg jump. This was once thought to be for the physician's amusement, but now we know that it is to test the patient's reflex arc. In the reflex arc shown in Figure elsewhere in this chapter, the impulse is generated in a special receptor called a *stretch receptor* that responds when it is elongated.

The impulse is then transmitted to a sensory neuron, which enters the spinal column over the *dorsal nerve root*. The impulse is then transferred to the proper motor neuron. The motor neuron leaves the spinal cord over the *ventral nerve root* and travels outward to the effector, a muscle group.

In most other reflex arcs the impulse is transmitted from sensory to motor neurons by an *association neuron*. (The system of association neurons can be so complex that the circuit is no longer considered a reflex arc.) Note that *impulses* from one side of the body can cross the spinal cord so that effectors in the other side of the body are stimulated.

In addition, the incoming impulse can be transmitted to the *dendrites* of yet other neurons, *ascending neurons*, which go up the spinal cord to the brain. In this way, even if the response has already been accomplished reflexively, the brain is informed of the change. Direct neural routing from the spinal cord in a *reflex arc* saves time because the distance the impulse has to travel from receptor to effector is shorter. Furthermore, no time is spent in *deliberating* over the decision.

We have considered the brain and spinal cord in the simplest of terms, but even so, the complexity of this great central nervous system becomes apparent. As more of its mysteries are solved even more intriguing questions are revealed. It gives up its secrets slowly, but *researchers* continue to probe at the central nervous system with the greatest tool of all, their own.

Many of the brain's precise *mechanisms* remain a mystery. And while we often do not understand just how the brain is affected by *various* chemicals, we are often keenly aware of their results. So, let's briefly consider some of the more common means of chemically altering brain function and behaviour.

The Vertebrate Brain

Actually, there is no such thing as the vertebrate brain, because the *vertebrates* include widely diverse groups, each of which is highly *specialised* and *distinctive*. In the midst of such diversity, however, it is possible to detect trends that give some clues to the general pattern of brain development in animals with *backbones*.

Figure elsewhere in this chapter illustrates relative differences in parts of the brain from fish to reptile to bird to *mammal*. The *medulla* is the part of the brain that connects directly with the spinal cord allowing messages to be transmitted between the brain and the rest of the body. In addition, it controls vital functions such as *breathing* and *heart rate*. The *cerebellum* is associated with sensory motor coordination for locomotion and posture.

The cerebrum is the "*gray matter*," the thinking part of the brain. (Regarding the brain, the higher centers are those most recently evolved advanced"—and usually refer to the *cerebrum*. The lower centers are more ancient—"primitive"—and generally refer to areas nearer the medulla.) We will discuss all these structures shortly, but there are a few *preliminary* points you might find interesting.

We might note for example that, not only is there an increase in general brain size (in relation to body size and, particularly, to *spinal cord* size) as we go from fish to mammal, but there is also an increase in the size of the cerebrum in relation to other parts of the brain. However, there are notable exceptions to this trend. For example, the olfactory lobe doesn't follow this pattern.

Olfaction has to do with the sense of smell, so which of the animals in Figure elsewhere in this chapter do you suppose would rely more on a *sense* of smell? (Remember to consider the olfactory lobe in relation to total brain size.) Other sensory lobes could also be singled out, such as the optic lobe, which has to do with vision. Which animal do you suppose would have a larger *optic lobe* with respect to its brain mass, an eagle or an elephant?

The fact that the cerebrum is larger as we move to more recently evolved (advanced) animals does not imply that as one moves up the evolutionary family tree, each species is "smarter" than the ones below it. There may be such a trend toward higher intelligence within certain groups, but there are also many exceptions.

For example, the octopus, a mollusk like the snail, is more intelligent than many vertebrates. In fact, the octopus brain is similar to the mammalian brain in terms of its complexity and organisation.

The evolutionary development of the mammalian cerebrum, which culminates in the human brain, *undoubtedly* has been one of the most *crucial* events in the history of life on earth. Such a statement is *admittedly* somewhat *grandiose*, but its validity becomes apparent when we consider the impact of the human species on the *fragile* life-support system that so thinly covers the planet. It would be interesting, therefore,

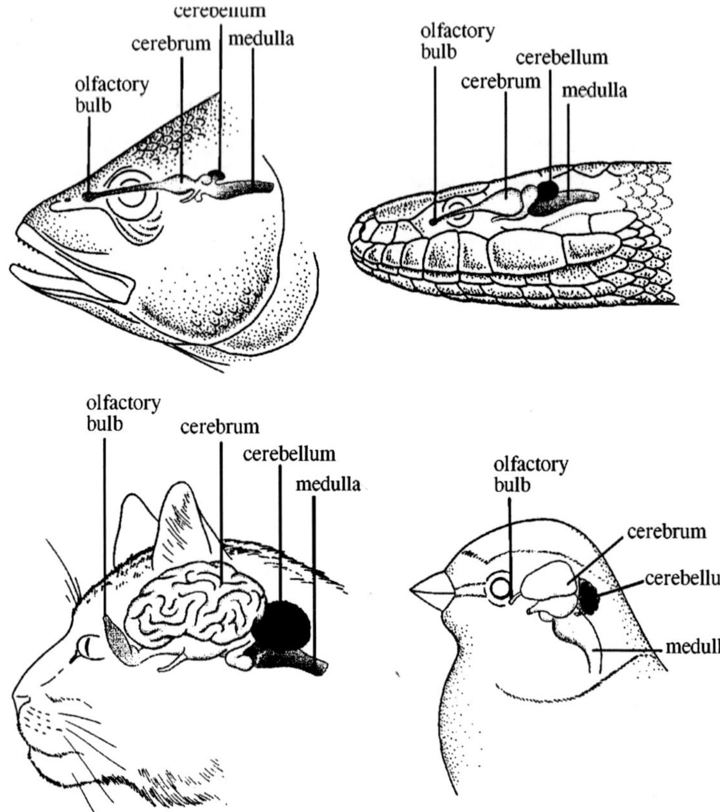

Figure 7.2 : A comparison of the brains of a fish, a reptile, a bird, and a mammal. Notice the diminutive size of the cerebrum relative to the olfactory bulb in the fish.

to know how such a brain came to be. What spurred its development? No one is certain, but one prevailing idea is that an increasingly developed cerebrum aided in the survival of one small *seemingly* insignificant group of reptiles that lived in an exceedingly dangerous world dominated by the great *dinosaurs*. This group, which was to give rise to mammals, branched off from other reptiles 180-200 million years ago.

These small premammals were certainly no match for the speedy, *incredibly* powerful, and voracious dinosaurs. Since they couldn't *outrun* or outfight the "*ruling reptiles*," it is believed that a *premium* was placed on their mental agility. In order to survive, the premammals were forced to outthink the dinosaurs. The dimmer members among them would rapidly have fallen to *predators* and, thus, would have failed to leave their "*dim genes*" in the next generation. So, with their very existence at stake, the premammals must have rapidly increased their mental agility, starting the cerebrum on its way toward dominating the brain of at least one line of animals.

The rapid development of the cerebrum and increasing reliance on intelligence would have been accompanied by other changes among the early mammals. For example, since learning requires experience, the brainier animals would have had to develop a life pattern that gave them a chance to learn before they were exposed to the dangers of the world. On this basis, some believe, parental care developed.

Even today the offspring of "*learning animals*" stay with their parents for extended periods. (How old were you when you left home?) During this time, they are cared for and protected by their parents until they gain enough experience to cope with the world. Also, by associating with parents or others of their kind, they can learn from them. (Most of the more brainy species are social animals, although there are notable exceptions.)

Even in a high-risk world, however, increased braininess is not the only course open to natural selection. As an example of another evolutionary route, consider the "*strategy*" of birds. The noted *psychologist Oscar Heinroth* is said to have commented, "Birds are so stupid because they can fly." The idea is that a bird doesn't normally "*outfox*" its enemies through intellectual maneuvering. It simply flies away.

Even in escaping airborne predators, such as hawks, most birds do not rely on their *cunning*. Instead, they employ a few *stereotyped* behaviour patterns, such as attacking in mass, aggregating to confuse predators, taking rather specific evasive *maneuvers*, or giving warning cries. Birds just never have had to develop great mental *capacities*, so don't be misled by the *discerning* frown on an eagle's face.

THE HUMAN BRAIN

Now we come to the rather interesting notion of the human brain talking about itself. Perhaps it is because of this strange twist that we encounter so many endless *accolades* about this great organ. Let's begin with some basic descriptions.

The human brain is divided into three parts: the hindbrain, the midbrain, and the forebrain. The *hindbrain* consists of the medulla, the cerebellum, and the pons. The hindbrain is sometimes called the "old brain" because it evolved first. These structures still dominate the brain of some animals, as we have seen. The *midbrain*, logically enough, is

Table 7.2 : Structuere and Function of Human Brain.

Structure	*Function*
Hindbrain	
medulla	Control of subconscious activities such as breathing, digestion, heartbeat, swallowing, vomiting, and sneezing; connects the spinal cord with the brain
cerebellum	Controls balance, equilibrium, and coordinaton
pons	Connects the cerebellum and the cerebral cortex
Midbrain	Connects the hindbrain and forebrain; receives sensory input from the eyes
Forebrain	
thalamus	The "great relay station;" connects various parts of brain
reticular system	Arousal of certain brain areas; filters impulses from sensory neurons
hypothalamus	Regulates heart rate, blood pressure, body temperature and the pituitary; controls drives such as hunger, thirst and sex
cerebrum	
cerebral cortex (outer cerebrum)	Gray matter, conscious thought; memory, intelligence, speech; association among senses
occipital lobe	Processes visual information
temporal lobe	Auditory reception and some visual information,
frontal lobe	Regulates precise voluntary movement and the use of language and speech (includes the prefrontal lobe, which sorts information and orders stimuli)
parietal lobe	Receives information from the skin and processes information about body position
white matter (inner cerebrum)	Nerve tracts allowing communication between parts of cortex; e.g. corpus callosum connects the two hemispheres and helps them communicate

the area between the forebrain and hindbrain and connects the two. The *forebrain*, or "*new brain*," consists of the two cerebral hemispheres and certain internal structures. Table elsewhere in this chapter summarises the structure and function of the parts of the brain.

The Hindbrain

The Medulla

As a rough *generality*, the more *subconscious*, or *mechanical*, processes are directed by the more posterior parts of the brain. For example, the hindmost part, the medulla, is specialised as a control center for such basic functions as breathing, digestion, and heartbeat. In addition, it is an important center of control for certain charming activities such as *swallowing*, *vomiting*, and *sneezing*. As we have already seen, it connects the spinal cord and the more anterior parts of the brain.

The Cerebellum and Pons

Above the medulla and more toward the back of the head is the *cerebellum*, which is concerned with balance, equilibrium, and coordination. Do you suppose there might be differences between athletes and nonathletes in this part of the brain? (Apparently, there are, but the differences are slight.)

Do you think this "*lower*" center of the brain is subject to modification through learning? (Can you improve your coordination through practice?) The *pons*, which is the portion of the brainstem just above the medulla, connects the cerebellum and the *cerebral cortex*, accenting the relationship between the cerebellar part of the hindbrain and the more "*conscious*" centers of the forebrain.

The Midbrain

The *midbrain* connects the hindbrain and forebrain by numerous tracts. In addition, certain parts of the midbrain receive sensory input from the eyes and ear. In vertebrates, sound is processed here before being sent to the forebrain. The midbrain has a more complex role in fishes and amphibians than in reptiles, birds, and mammals because in the latter group, many of its functions are taken over by the forebrain.

The Forebrain

The Thalamus and Reticular System

The thalamus and hypothalamus are located at the base of the forebrain. The *thalamus* is rather unpoetically called the "great relay station" of the brain. It consists of densely packed clusters of nervous cells that presumably connect the various parts of the brain-between the forebrain and the hindbrain, between different parts of the forebrain, and between parts of the sensory system and the cerebral cortex.

The thalamus contains a peculiar neural structure called the *reticular system*, an area of *interconnected neurons* that are almost feltlike in appearance. These neurons run throughout the *thalamus* and into the midbrain. The role of the reticular system is still a bit *mysterious*, but several interesting facts are known about it. For example, it bugs your brain. Every afferent and efferent pathway to and from the brain sends side branches to the *reticular* system as it passes through the *thalamus*. So all the brain's incoming and outgoing communications are "*tapped*." Also, these *reticular* neurons are rather unspecific.

That is, the same neuron may respond to stimuli from, say, the hand, foot, ear, or eye. It has been suggested that the reticular system serves to activate the appropriate parts of the brain upon receiving a stimulus. In other words, it acts as an arousal system for certain brain areas. Furthermore, the more messages it intercepts, the more the brain is aroused.

Thus, the reticular system is important to sleep. You may have noticed it is much easier to fall asleep lying on a soft bed in a quiet, darkened room than on a pool table in a disco. With the quietness, there are fewer incoming *stimuli*; as a result, the reticular system receives fewer messages and the brain is lulled rather than aroused. On those nights when you have the "*big eye*" and just can't sleep, the cause may be continued (possibly spontaneous) firing of reticular neurons.

The reticular system may also regulate which impulses are allowed to register in your brain. When you are *engrossed* in a television program, you may not notice that someone has entered the room. But when you are engaged in even more absorbing activities, it might take a general stimulus on the order of an *earthquake* to distract you, whereas the specific stimulus of a turning *doorknob* would immediately attract your attention. Such *filtering* and selective depression of stimuli apparently takes place in the reticular system.

The Hypothalamus

The *hypothalamus* is a small body, densely packed with cells. It helps regulate the internal environment as well as some aspects of behaviour. For example, the *hypothalamus* helps to control heart rate, blood pressure, and body temperature.

It also plays a part in the regulation of the pituitary gland, as we learned earlier. And it controls such basic drives as hunger, thirst, and sex. So now you know what to blame for all your problems. Experimental electrical stimulation of various centers in the hypothalamus can cause a cat to act *hungry*, *angry*, *cold*, *hot*, *benign*, or *horny*.

The Cerebrum

For many people the word *brain conjures* up an image of two large, deeply convoluted gray lobes. What they have in mind, of course, is the outside layer of the two cerebral hemispheres, the dominant physical aspect of the *human brain*. The cerebrum is present in all vertebrates, but it assumes particular importance in humans. In some animals, it is essentially an elaborate refinement that implements behaviour that could be performed to some degree without it.

It has a far greater importance in other animals. For example, if the cerebral cortex of a frog is removed, the frog will show relatively little change in behaviour *(cortex,* rind; the cerebral cortex is the outer layer of the forebrain in which a great deal of the active neural tissue is found). If the frog is turned upside down, it will right itself; if it is touched with an irritant, it will scratch; it will even catch a fly.

Also, sexual behaviour in frogs can occur without the use of the brain—but we'll try not to extrapolate from that. Rats, on the other hand, are more dependent on their cerebral cortex. A rat that is surgically deprived of its cerebrum can visually distinguish only light and dark, although its body movement seems unimpaired.

A decorticated cat (that is, with its cerebral cortex removed) can *meow*, *purr*, *swallow*, and move to avoid pain, but its movements are *sluggish* and robotlike. A monkey whose cerebral cortex has been removed is severely paralyzed and can barely distinguish light and dark. In humans, the destruction of the cortex causes total blindness and almost complete paralysis. Although such persons can breathe and swallow, they soon die.

It seems apparent that the cerebrum is more than just the center of "*intelligence*," and that from an evolutionary standpoint, as the cerebrum enlarges, more and more of the functions of the lower brain are transferred to it.

Hemispheres and Lobes

The human cerebrum consists of two hemispheres, the left and the right, each of these being divided into four lobes. At the back is the *occipital lobe*, which receives and analyzes visual information.

The *temporal lobe* is at the side of the brain. It roughly resembles the thumb on a boxing glove, and it is bounded anteriorly by the *fissure of Sylvius*. The temporal lobe shares in the processing of visual information, but its main function is auditory reception.

The *frontal lobe* is right where you would expect to find it-at the front of the cerebrum, just behind the forehead. This is the part that people hit with the heel of the palm when they suddenly remember what they forgot. One part of the *frontal* lobe is the center for the regulation of precise voluntary movement. Another part functions importantly in the use of language, and damage here results in speech *impairment*. The area at the very front of the frontal lobe is called the *prefrontal area*, if you follow that.

Whereas it was once believed that this area was the seat of intellect, it is now apparent that its principal function is sorting out information and ordering *stimuli*. In other words, it places information and stimuli into their proper context. The gentle touch of a mate or the sight of a hand protruding from the bathtub drain might both serve as stimuli, but they would be *sorted* differently by the prefrontal area.

Up until a few years ago, parts of the frontal lobe were surgically removed in efforts to bring the behaviour of certain aberrant individuals more into line with what *psychologists* had decided was the norm. The operation was called a frontal lobotomy, and it resulted in passive and *unimaginative* individuals. Fortunately, the practice has been largely discontinued, largely because chemical treatments now meet the same objectives.

The *parietal lobe* lies directly behind the frontal lobe and is separated from it by the *fissure of Rolando*. This lobe receives stimuli from the skin receptors, and it helps to process information regarding bodily position. Even if you can't see your feet right now, you have some idea of where they are thanks to receptors in the parietal lobe. Damage to the parietal lobe may produce *numbness* and may cause a person to perceive his or her own body as wildly *distorted* and to be unable to perceive spatial relationships in the environment.

By probing the brain with electrodes, it has been possible to determine exactly which area of the cerebrum is involved in the body's various sensory and *motor activities*. We can see the results of such *mapping* in the rather grotesque Figure elsewhere in this chpater. The pictures are distorted not out of any appreciation of the *macabre*, but to demonstrate that the area of the cerebrum devoted to each body part is dependent not on the size of the part, but on the importance it has come to have in the natural history of humans.

Thus, we have the greatest number of sensory receptors in the face, hands, and genitals, but the greatest amount of control only in the face and hands (as you may have already discovered). Such probing has also revealed that memories are stored in very specific places.

Also note that the sensory and motor areas are not randomly scattered through the cortex, but that proximity in brain areas reflects the *proximity* of the parts of the body they control. Thus the index finger control area lies near the thumb control area, and the *elbow* area lies closer to the finger area than does the shoulder area.

Two Brains, Two Minds?

The best way to begin a banal conversation a few years ago was, "What sign are you?" Today, though, *sophisticates* may lead with, "Are you right brained or left brained?" Some of the findings of one of the most fascinating branches of neural research has indeed filtered into the public *consciousness*.

The question is based on information that has been *accumulating* since the middle of the last century when A. L. Wigam, a British physician, performed autopsies on men who had led normal lives with only half a brain. That is, one *hemisphere* had been destroyed by accident or other trauma. The question then arose, since we only need half a brain, then, why do we have two?

At first it was assumed that this was another case where nature had built in *redundancy*, or backup, in a *critical* system. Brain research has revealed a fascinating fact: the hemispheres are not duplicates at all, but structures with quite different *specialisations*. To oversimplify, the left hemisphere is the center of logical, stepwise reasoning, of mathematics and language.

It processes information in a *fragmentary*, *sequential* manner, *sorting* out the parts of questions and dealing with each quite rationally. (*Star Trek's* Spock was definitely left brained.) The right brain, on the other hand, is the center of awareness for music and art. Imagination swells from this lobe and it sees things in their entirety (*holistically*), often solving problems through *insight*, as it compares relationships.

The flexibility of the two *hemispheres* has been shown when one is damaged and the other takes over its role. Such *flexibility*, by the way, may be greater in left handers than in right handers. It seems that the brain centers of *southpaws* are generally more diffuse, less localised, with functions more equally dispersed between the two *hemispheres*. Brain damage to left handers may produce different symptoms than right handers with similar *injuries*.

The two halves of the brain are connected by a great, broad tract, about 4 inches wide [called the *corpus callosum*]. Information from each half can be *communicated* to the other half via the corpus *callosum*. Thus, special abilities of the two parts of the brain can be *integrated* and we are able to solve problems, perform tasks, and appreciate life's offerings by a grand union of complex and differing abilities.

Or maybe not. Evidence indicates that usually one hemisphere is dominant and inordinately influences how we approach life. Furthermore, some researchers argue that the hemispheres somehow compete with each other for our attention. Such arguments, at this point, quickly extend beyond science and enter the realm of the *philosopher*.

The Split Brain

If we learn a visual *discrimination* (such as correct and incorrect shapes) with one eye covered, we can make the same discrimination with the other eye. Anatomically, the reason is because fibers from the inner (medial) halves of each eye cross over the *optic chiasma* to the other side of the brain, as shown in Figure elsewhere in this chapter.

Thus, the visual centers in both halves of the cerebrum receive information from both eyes. If the *optic chiasma* is split, the right eye can still make the same *discriminations* as the left, and vice versa. However, the brain halves are joined by a flattened band called the corpus callosum.

If the corpus *callosum* is also split, then things learned by using one eye remain unknown to the other side of the brain. Nothing learned by one half of the brain is transferred to the other half. This means, in effect, that mammals have two brains that can act *independently*. In fact, it is possible to train both halves of the brain separately.

A split-brain monkey can be trained to approach an object if it is seen with one eye and to withdraw from the same object if it is seen with the other eye. If the monkey sees the object with both eyes, however, usually one side of the brain will take over and the monkey will respond without hesitation by either approaching or withdrawing.

THE PERIPERAL NERVOUS SYSTEM

Pairs of thick, white nerves emerge from the brain and spinal cord and innervate every receptor and effector in the entire body. These nerves comprise the *peripheral nervous system*.

Those nerves (12 pairs in humans) extending from the brain are called the *cranial nerves*. Further down, the spinal cord gives rise to thick spinal nerves (31 pairs in humans). Each nerve is formed from the union of a dorsal and ventral nerve root that emerge directly from the spinal cord.

The *dorsal nerve root* (comprised of sensory neurons) is swollen by a huge ganglion at about the level where it enters the spinal column. The ganglion houses the cell bodies of all the sensory neurons entering the spinal column. The cell bodies of the neurons comprising the *ventral nerve root* (comprised of motor neurons) lie embedded in the spinal column, so these nerves are not disfigured by ganglia. The two great nerves fuse just outside the spinal column and travel together for a way before giving rise to increasingly smaller nerves-nerves that will ultimately branch into delicate neurons that reach every part of the body.

The peripheral nervous system consists of the somatic nervous system and the *autonomic* nervous system. The somatic nervous system carries the impulses that we are most conscious of, the commands to our voluntary muscles and the conscious sensations from all parts of our bodies. The autonomic nervous system is more concerned with our conscious and involuntary internal workings.

The Autonomic Nervous System

The autonomic nervous system is formed from a special set of peripheral nerves that serve the heart, lungs, digestive tract, and other internal organs. This system is largely under the control of the *hypothalamus*.

The autonomic nervous system can be divided into the *sympathetic* and *parasympathetic nervous systems*, which act antagonistically. If the sympathetic system works to speed up certain body processes, then the parasympathetic system works to slow them down, and vice versa.

The sympathetic nervous system is activated in what has been called "*fight-or-flight*" reactions. It also functions in reproductive behaviour, but perhaps we should avoid further *alliteration*. The fight-or-flight syndrome becomes apparent in certain emergency situations. For example, if a bear rushes into the room where you are quietly reading, your body will react "*sympathetically.*"

The pupils of your eyes will dilate, the better to see the bear; blood vessels to the brain and skeletal muscles will increase in diame-ter, bringing oxygen-laden blood to these structures; the better to plan and effect your escape. Peripheral blood vessels will decrease in diameter, so blood loss will be minimised in case the bear swats you on your way out; heart rate will increase, bringing oxygen to your running muscles; and *digestion* will almost stop, since your blood is needed elsewhere. So much blood may go to your muscles that your blood supply to the brain may decrease, causing you to faint, in which case you will hope the bear is just there as part of some effort to help curb forest fires.

If upon awakening, you should discover the bear was only your *roommate* in a bear suit, your parasympathetic system will take over and reverse all these responses. You may then wish to activate the sympathetic system of your roommate.

Whereas the parasympathetic nervous system brings about its effects with the neurotransmitter *acetylcholine*, the sympathetic nervous system

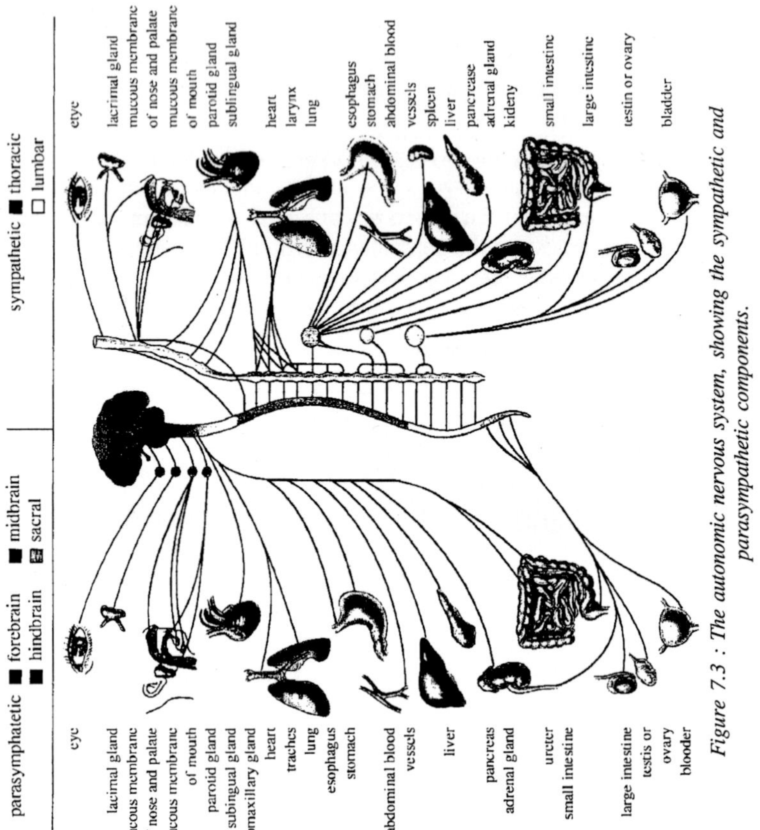

Figure 7.3 : The autonomic nervous system, showing the sympathetic and parasympathetic components.

causes its effects with the transmitter substance *epinephrine* (*adrenaline*). You might wonder why *epinephrine* couldn't simply be released from the adrenal glands in an emergency situation, to travel in the blood and elicit these same changes throughout the body-why it is necessary to develop another, but similar, emergency system.

Actually, the adrenal gland may secrete adrenaline into the *bloodstream* in such a stress situation, but the two emergency reactions (a *general* one, as the adrenal gland alerts the entire system, and a specific one, in which certain nerves activate only specific areas) illustrate the important difference between hormonal and neural regulation.

The sympathetic system releases its adrenaline *directly* into the proper effector. Only small amounts are released, so although the response is immediate, it is of short duration. Greater amounts of *adrenaline* may be secreted by the adrenal gland, and while these take longer to reach the effector, their effect is more long-lasting. As was pointed out earlier, then, neural regulation is more immediate and short-term than hormonal regulation.

Autonomic Learning

The *autonomic* nervous system is usually described as "*involuntary.*" It is assumed that we do not normally exercise *conscious* control over its functions. While it is true that the autonomic system can, and normally does, function in the absence of conscious control, there is evidence that some conscious control is possible. In other words, we may be able to learn to *influence* some of our autonomic reactions.

L. V. Dicara and N. E. Miller of Rockefeller University were able to teach rats to increase or decrease heart rate, blood pressure, intestinal contractions, blood vessel diameter, and even rate of urine formation. They did this by monitoring the animals normal patterns and *fluctuations* in these parameters over a period of time.

As natural variations occurred, the ones in the desired direction were rewarded by electrical stimulation of the "*pleasure center*" of the brain; variations in the other direction were punished by a slight but unpleasant shock. For example, if the experimenter wanted the rat to learn to slow its heart rate, when the heart slowed naturally, the animal would be rewarded; when it accelerated naturally, punishment would follow. Soon the heart beat more slowly.

The researchers produced similar results in humans and have even taught some to control their blood pressure.

The possible applications of autonomic learning are quite varied and fascinating. For example, some of the amazing *feats* accomplished by some practitioners of yoga, such as when they drastically lower their *metabolic* rate, may be due to *autonomic* learning. In other cases, autonomic learning can aid in survival against the elements.

It is known, for example, that *mountain* people of the *Himalayas*, such as the famed Sherpa guides, are able to withstand extreme cold. They may show no effects from sleeping barefoot in the frigid mountains. It has been suggested that such feats are possible because they have "*learned*" to withdraw body fluids from their extremities so that cell membranes cannot be ruptured by the formation of ice crystals.

Some have suggested that autonomic learning has not received the attention it deserves in the Western world. However, a *phenomenon* known as *biofeedback* has received a good deal of attention, especially among harried professionals who see themselves caught up in the *frenzy* of the rat race, Here, people are taught to monitor their *brainwave* activity in order to consciously provided with information that allows them to monitor their autonomic processes and control them. For example, when given information on their brainwaves, they may learn to consciously generate those waves that indicate *restfulness* and *peace.*

MINDBENDERS

For some reason, a lot of people don't seem to like the minds they were born with. A great deal of our energy, it seems, is spent in finding ways to "*bend*" our minds and change our moods. And (in spite of popular beliefs) the search is not a new one. With all the profound problems facing our ancestors, they almost immediately set about learning to make booze. Also, we find hallucinogens were important in many of our earliest known cultures.

The search for mindbenders continues today, however, in ways our ancestors could only imagine. (The ancient Greeks, for example, were not big on sniffing transmission fluid.) So some of the things we will mention here have been with us for ages, while others are so new that we really don't know how they act or what their long-term effects are.

We can begin by noting that "*drugs*" are *psychoactive agents*. That is, they can alter mood, memory, attention, control, judgment, time—and space sense, emotion, and sensation. Fortunately, probably none do all of these at once. Most cause effects that can be placed along a continuum between *stimulation* (an excitatory state) and *depression* (a state of reduced mental activity).

Here, we will review a few general principles about a few of the major groups. Not unexpectedly, we will find that all have potential for abuse. Table elsewhere in this chapter lists a few mindbending drugs and their effects on the human body.

Abuse may arise because of our tendencies to overdo the drug or to overly rely on the drugs. Use of some drugs can cause *dependence* or *addiction*. There are two major forms of drug dependence. *Physical dependence* occurs when the drug is necessary simply to maintain bodily comfort. It's disuse causes sometimes agonizing discomfort (called *withdrawal symptoms*). *Psychological dependence* exists where a drug is necessary for mental or emotional comfort. Withdrawal symptoms here can be as severe as they are for physical dependence.

Tobacco

Tobacco is the dried leaf of the plant *Nicotiana tabacum*. It is usually rolled, *shredded*, or flaked and then burned. The smoke is inhaled, allowing its products to cross the thin-walled alveoli of the

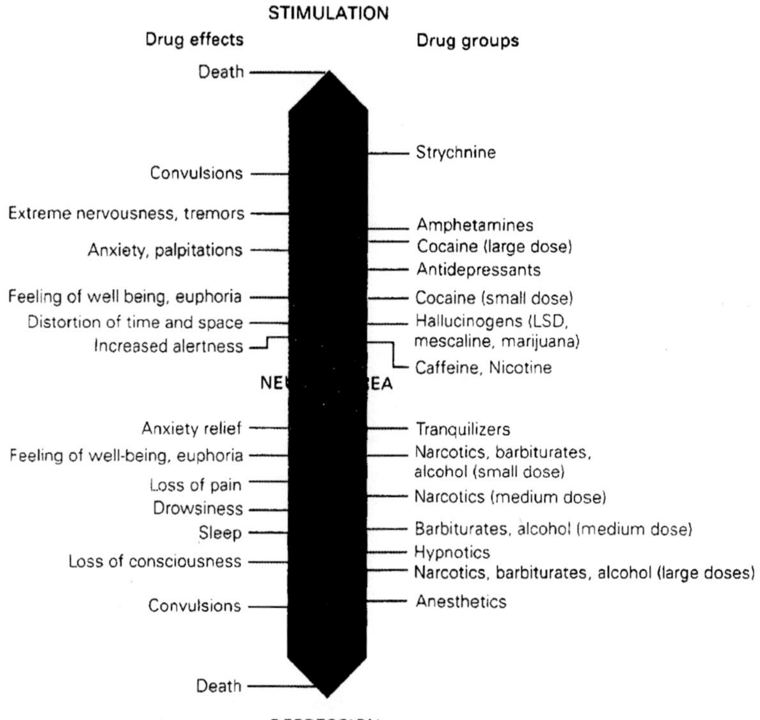

Figure 7.4 : A continuum of drug action. The effects are shown at left, the various agents at right. The neutral area is drug-free.

lungs and to enter the bloodstream. Over 6,800 different chemicals are found in tobacco smoke, many of them carcinogens (cancer-causers).

There is evidence that the major psychoactive product *nicotine* is carcinogenic. In large doses, nicotine may also cause *cramps*, *vomiting*, *diarrhea*, *dizziness*, *confusion*, and *tremors*. It can cause respiratory failure and death, the ultimate lesson.

The poison is particularly dangerous to nonsmokers who have not developed a. tolerance to nicotine. For them 75 milligrams of nicotine could *threaten* life (that is, the amount in about 3.5 packs of *cigarettes*). The development of the smoking habit is *curious* because the first attempts can be *ghastly*. Perhaps, though, its continuance is even more curious because smoking has been clearly linked to lung cancer, *emphysema*, heart and *circulatory ailments*, and birth defects. (It also contributes to premature aging of the skin.)

Nevertheless, we continue to be susceptible to advertising touting

Table 7.3 : Some Mindbending Drugs.

Drug	*Action*	*Effects/Risks*	*Dependence*	*Tolerance*
Tobacco	stimulant	causes lung cancer and emphysema; heart and blood vessel damage	physical and psychological	
Caffeine	stimulant	increases alertness; increases heart rate and blood pressure high doses cause irritability and nervousness	some degree of psychological	with large amounts
THC (Marijuana/ Hashish)	low dose is similar to sedative; high dose similar to hallucinogen	smoke causes lung damage; mild euphoria; THC accumulates in fatty tissues	no; possibly slight psychological	no
Alcohol	depressant	euphoria; loss of motor coordination (high dose); slows reflexes; damage to liver, stomach, intestines, damage to nerve cells; damage to heart and skeletal muscle	physical and psychological	develops quickly
Opiates	depressant	euphoria; drowsiness & sleep; muscle relaxation	strong physical	

Table Contd.

Drug	*Action*	*Effects/Risks*	*Dependence*	
Cocaine	stimulant	euphoria; increased energy; increased heart rate and blood pressure	physical and psychological (especially with crack)	little
Amphetamines	stimulant	increased energy; alertness; decreased appetite	physical and psychological	yes
Barbiturates	depressant	reduced anxiety; sleep	high potential for physical	yes, increases rapidly
Phencylidine	anesthetic; psychedelic	euphoria; relaxation psychosis; violence; coma	?	?
Methaqualone	depressant	reduced anxiety; relaxation drowsiness & sleep	physical	increases rapid
Psychedelics	psychedelic	hallucinations; distortion of time, space and sensation; "bad trips"	no physical; possible psychological	yes

the blessings of smoking. Smoke can permanently paralyze the tiny cilia that sweep the breathing passages clean and can cause the lining of the respiratory tract to thicken irregularly. The body's attempt to rid itself of the smoking toxins may produce a deep, hacking cough in the person next to you at the lunch counter.

Console yourself with the knowledge that these hackers are only trying to rid their bodies of nicotines, "*tars*," *formaldehyde*, *hydrogen sulfide*, *resins*, and who knows what. lust enjoy your meal.

Smoking may cause physiological dependence on the products in the smoke. Withdrawal may produce a variety of unpleasant reactions, and some people are apparently unable to stop, no matter what the results. The American Cancer Society estimates that about 90 percent of all lung cancer (which has a low cure-rate and which is now the number one cause of cancer deaths) is due to smoking and that if smoking ceased, the incidence of all cancers in the U.S. would fall about 25-30 percent. (You should be aware that so-called "*smokeless* tobacco," such as snuff or chewing plugs, has also been linked to cancer, especially of the mouth.)

Caffeine

Caffeine is a component of coffee, tea, chocolate, and many colas. Caffeine is a stimulant, affecting the central nervous system. It works by stimulating nerve cell metabolism. Such drinks were not always so popular. In fact, at one time in the Near East, *coffee* drinkers were put to death-perhaps, some would say, a fate not worse than having to start the day without coffee.

Caffeine increases alertness and decreases fatigue and boredom. It also speeds the heart rate, increases blood pressure, increases urine formation, and dilates some blood vessels while contracting others. In small to moderate amounts (two to four cups), it may improve performance in boring or repetitive tasks, but it does not help in more complex intellectual tasks, such as reading or doing long division.

However, it may help keep you awake so you can perform those tasks, since it inhibits sleep. In higher doses, it causes nervousness, irritability, and a "*jangled*" feeling. Very high doses can cause convulsions, but you would have to drink about 100 cups before you run a risk of dying. (By then, you probably would have already talked yourself to death.)

People who consume very large amounts of coffee, say ten to twenty cups a day, may develop *caffeinism*. The symptoms are *insomnia*, high blood pressure, increased body temperature, racing heart, and chills. (Caffeine is also known to encourage the development of breast cysts in women.)

One develops *tolerance* for caffeine so that increasingly higher doses are needed to produce the same effect. Withdrawal symptoms include *headaches* and *irritability*. Withdrawing coffee drinkers are generally not considered dangerous.

Marijuana and Hashish (THC)

Marijuana (also known as dope, pot, grass, reefer, killer weed, or Mary Jane) is a form of Indian hemp *(Cannabis sativa)*, and was cultivated in the United States during World War II to produce fibers for ropes after the supply of hemp from the *Philippines* was cut off. The wild progeny of those plants has driven *crusading* law *enforcement* officers up the wall, and the attempt to control the drug continues to absorb *enormous* amounts of public money.

The active ingredient in marijuana is a group of chemicals called tetrahydrocannabinols (THC). Whereas marijuana users generally smoke the leaves (or eat them in brownies), THC is highest in a preparation called *hashish* (or *hash*), which is the concentrated resinous exudate collected from marijuana plants. Marijuana induces a mild *euphoria*, sometimes expressed as a happy or *giggly* mood.

It may also produce mild *hallucinations* (if there is such a thing), forgetfulness and reduce mental agility. Its effect varies among individuals and may be partly dependent upon the setting in which it is used. Some of the statements, official and otherwise, about marijuana have sometimes been ill-conceived, incorrect, and irrational. Because of the ludicrous nature of earlier official warnings about pot, there has been a tendency to reject all warnings regarding drugs. Perhaps this is unfortunate because marijuana can, indeed, produce problems.

For one thing, THC is fat-soluble and cannot be flushed out of the body by the kidneys. Instead it collects in the fatty tissues, such as the brain and reproductive organs. THC is slowly released as the fat is *metabolised*. Marijuana smoke is a powerful lung irritant and with regular use can cause not only bronchitis, but, apparently, precancerous changes in lung cells. (We must keep in mind that heavy marijuana use is a recent trend and it was only after sixty years of heavy cigarette smoking that its devastating effects became apparent.)

Other studies show that marijuana temporarily reduces sperm production and may cause the production of abnormal sperm. In female monkeys, it can disrupt *ovulation* and cause abnormal cycles. THC can cross the placenta in some laboratory animals and is associated with a higher rate of *miscarriages*. (It should definitely be avoided by pregnant women.) Marijuana is generally not considered addictive, and there seems to be little "*tolerance*," so doses need not be continuously increased.

There may be *psychological* "*dependence*" on the drug because of what the user regards as its rewarding effects. *Cannabis sativa* has been cultivated in the Near East for centuries. There, its THC is extracted to produce the resinous hashish. *Hashish* gets its name because it was used by the hashshashin, a Moslem terrorist group whose *notorious* violence was thought to be a result of addiction to the drug.

However, more careful studies of the hashshashin (the source of the word assassin), indicate that hashish was actually given as a reward for their murderous deeds-perhaps to produce the "*visions of glory*" promised by their leader, who, by the way, was a classmate of the poet Omar Khayyam.

Alcohol

Adolescent cynics have for years noted that while their parents were almost rabid in their opposition to other drugs, alcohol was often quite acceptable to them. The kids have a point. *Alcohol* is, indeed, a drug, even in the technical sense. And it is probably far more harmful than some of the drugs *alcoholics* fear.

The most immediate sign of its harmful effect is in the form of the hangover. No matter what the drink—beer, wine, or Singapore slings—the active ingredient is ethanol (CH_3CH_2OH). Ethanol, in spite of its reputation, is not a *stimulant*, it is a *depressant*. It may stimulate in a sense, however, because it can depress inhibitions and release the clever fellow within us all. It is also not an aphrodisiac, although it can in smaller amounts reduce anxieties.

In larger doses, it interferes with the sexual act in a most frustrating manner. As *Shakespeare* observed, it "*provokes* the desire, but it takes away the performance." People develop a tolerance for alcohol rather quickly. That is, as the body "*handles it*," more and more is required to produce the same effect. Essentially, the "*handling*" is mainly done by the liver, which can oxidise about an ounce of alcohol per hour. (Five to ten percent is excreted by the lungs and kidneys.)

Finally, though, the liver may become so damaged that it can *detoxify* very little alcohol. Alcohol is very addictive, and its use can produce severe withdrawal symptoms, the most drastic of which are delirium tremens, or DTs. Longterm use can damage the central and *peripheral* nervous systems, the liver, the *stomach*, and the *intestines*, but the effects vary greatly from one individual to the next.

One alcoholic's mind may go, while a drinking companion may only die of cirrhosis of the liver. Interestingly, heavy "binge" drinking may be safer than daily drinking of smaller amounts, perhaps because the layoffs give the liver time to recover.

Opiates

Opiates fall within the realm of what are referred to as "*hard drugs*." They are technically narcotics in that they depress the nervous system, and they can relieve pain and produce sleep or a *stupor*. The group includes *heroin*, *opium*, and *morphine*. Users rapidly develop tolerance, and continued use often results in addiction.

Consequently, the user not only needs the drug continually, but in increasingly higher doses. Because of the cost of opiates, addicts often resort to crime in order to finance their habit.

Injection of opiates produces a "*rush*," or sudden pleasurable sensation. (in beginners, it may also produce severe nausea.) The rush is followed by a great sense of well-being, accompanied by a marked decrease in physical drive. An accompanying drowsiness produces the nodding you can see in almost any New York subway.

Withdrawal symptoms following abrupt discontinuation of the drug are usually very violent. With heavy *addiction*, withdrawal may produce such an intense shock to the system that death results.

Cocaine

Cocaine (*toot*, *coke*, *lady*, *girl*) is another of those recently fashionable drugs that we don't know enough about. However, much of what we do know points to an *insidious* and potentially very *dangerous* substance. But, it was not always regarded so. In fact, it was once sold in the United States under its own name or used to lace other products, such as *Coca Cola*. It seems to stimulate neural activity in the brain by inhibiting the breakdown of *neurotransmitters*.

Cocaine is an alkaloid extract usually derived from two species of the *coca plant*, a South American shrub of the genus *Erythroxylon*. Historically, the leaves were chewed by pre-Columbian South American Indians, and the practice continues in that area to this day. The effect of chewing the leaves is a generally elevated intensity and an increase in apparent energy.

Today, however, chemical extraction techniques can produce a white, crystalline powder that is usually "*snorted*" (inhaled through the nose), "*shot*" (injected into veins), or "*based*" (where the alkaloid is chemically freed and smoked-"free basing"). *Snorting* cocaine produces the least *drastic* effects; basing produces the most powerful. In all cases there is a euphoria, mood elevation, and general stimulation. The result is talkativeness and a general intensity that may cause other people to tiptoe away.

As it wears off, a depression sets in that compels the user to seek another "*hit.*" The comedown from crack, a highly addictive and apparently inexpensive based form that is usually smoked, is severe that the user will do anything to avoid it.

The long term effects of regular cocaine use can be severe. The user may focus on the drug while other facets of life are neglected. The drug was once considered *physiologically nonaddictive*, but new evidence indicates that it can be powerfully addictive. There is little tolerance, so increasingly larger doses are not required.

Cocaine also has an artificially elevated expense. Whereas it costs only a few cents to manufacture a gram of cocaine, the street price may be $60 to $150. Furthermore, there may be little of the drug left in the street powder by the time it reaches the user. As a rule, it is "*stepped on*" (cut) by each person through whose hands it passes.

Amphetamines

Amphetamines, often loosely referred to as "*speed*" or "*uppers*," include a number of commercial drugs such as Benzedrine, *Dexedrine*, and *Methedrine*. Their chemical properties are similar to those of *epinephrine* that is, they cause great bursts of energy that can overcome feelings of fatigue.

Students and truck drivers have been known to take low doses in order to stay awake during midnight cramming sessions and long hauls, respectively. Weight watchers also use them to decrease appetite. Because *amphetamines* are effective in improving performance on *rigorous physical* tasks, they are sometimes used by athletes. Low doses do not impair skills or judgment.

A derivative called "*crystal meth*" (*methamphetamine*) is currently undergoing a resurgence on the street. The addition of a methyl group to the active molecule apparently makes for a smoother high. These people with an intense interest in the short term may use "*speed balls*", a mixture of *amphetamines* and *heroin*. The greatest abuse of amphetamines is by injection of the drug.

This produces an initial rush, followed by a feeling of *vigor* and euphoria that may last several hours. After this, however, come the dues. They appear in the form of *aching*, *discontent*, and *irritability*. To delay this letdown, the user may *boost* himself or herself with another injection. The high may thus last for days, during which time the user usually fails to eat or sleep. The end of this period may be followed by *exhaustion*, *severe depression*, *paranoia*, *aggressiveness*, *extreme irritability*, and *emotional* overreaction.

Users develop a tolerance for *amphetamines*, and *cessation* after prolonged use may produce withdrawal symptoms, although they are less severe than those associated with opiate withdrawal.

Barbiturates

Barbiturates, or "*downers*," are sold under a variety of trade names, including Nembutal, Seconal, Tuinal, and Amytal. They are all *sedativehypnotics* that act on the *cerebral* cortex, midbrain, and brainstem areas. Their effect is to reduce anxiety and induce *drowsiness* and sleep. These results are accompanied by loss of muscular coordination and slurring of speech, similar reactions to those induced by alcohol.

Barbiturates are highly addictive and rapidly produce tolerance. Withdrawal symptoms may be as severe as with *opiate* or *alcohol* withdrawal. The heavy *barbiturate* user is likely to be *confused*, *obnoxious*, *stubborn*, and *irritable*. In contrast to the *placid disinterest* of the opiate user, barbiturate users may be particularly *aggressive* and *violent*.

Barbiturates and alcohol acting together are particularly *dangerous*. The combination may cause death by suppressing the breathing centers. In addition, because each drug causes mental confusion, accidental deaths in those who mix them are all too common.

Phencylidine

Phencylidine, also called PCP or angel dust, is one of the more dangerous drugs to make the rounds in recent years, finding its place among certain *abysmally* ignorant young people. Unfortunately, many people use this powerful animal tranquilizer without realising it, since it is used to "*lace*" marijuana and even cocaine. Its users may feel euphoric and extremely relaxed, but the side effects of the drug include *extreme violence*, *psychosis*, *confusion*, and, at high *doses*, *coma*.

Methaqualone

Methaqualone (Quaalude, or lude) is a synthetic *barbiturate*. When it was introduced in 1963, it was believed to be *nonaddictive* and was prescribed freely. However, all this has changed; it is indeed addictive. It often causes the user to be relaxed, uninhibited, and receptive (as a result it has been touted as an *aphrodisiac*). When taken with *alcohol*, one may fall into a stupor ("*lude out*") and lose control of movement. This is accompanied by a feeling of "*pins and needles*" in the extremities and around the mouth.

Psychedelics

Psychedelics are comprised of a group of drugs that produce hallucinations and various other phenomena that very closely mimic certain mental disorders. These drugs include lysergic acid diethylamide (LSD), *mescaline*, *peyote*, *psilocybin*, and various commercial preparations such as Sernyl and Ditran.

Of these, LSD is probably the best known. Although its use has apparently diminished since its heyday in the late 1960s, it seems to be making a comeback in some special circles. LSD is synthesized from lysergic acid produced by a fungus (*ergot*) that is parasitic on cereal grains such as rye.

It usually produces responses in a particular sequence. The initial reactions may include *weakness*, *dizziness*, and *nausea*. These symptoms are followed by a distortion of time and space. The senses may become intensified and *strangely* intertwined-that is, sounds can be "*seen*" and colours "*heard*."

Finally, there may be changes in mood, a feeling of separation of the self from the *framework* of time and space, and changes in the *perception* of the self. The *sensations* experienced under the influence of psychedelics are unlike anything encountered within the normal range of experiences. The descriptions of users therefore can only be *puzzling* to nonusers. Some users experience bad trips or "*bummers*," which have been known to produce long-term effects. Bad trips can be *terrifying* experiences and can occur in experienced users for no apparent reason.

Our nervous systems are the products of natural selection, and so they are specialised to help us deal successfully with the part of the world with which humans must interact. We see, though, that various aspects of our psyches can be satisfied, and perceived "*needs*" can be met, by a wide range of chemicals that our natural bodies are not prepared to deal with.

Some of these chemicals have been around so long that they, and their dangers, have become familiar-even accepted. Others, though, are new, and we await data on the effects of their long-term use. And we are an inventive species, so we must assume that other "*mindbenders*" lie just over the horizon—new chemicals, new experiences, new behaviours, and new dangers.

8

THE SENSES

What kind of world is this and how do we know? It seems obvious that whatever we know, we know through our senses. Immediately, however, this answer brings us into difficulties. This is partly because our senses *monitor* only certain aspects of the environment, so what about those things we can't detect? Aren't they, too, part of our world?

If you were to ask a variety of animals to describe what the earth is like, there would be little *consensus*. A fly might describe swirling eddies, delicious surfaces, and a *kaleidoscopic* world of *shimmering mosaics*. A bee would see deep violet colours in flowers that we call yellow, while the red rose would appear to be black, lacking colour at all.

A dog might describe a gray, drab world *dominated* by surges of sounds, accented by *thundering* odours. A *tapeworm* might speak vaguely of a warm, wet world preceded by harsh light and *withering dryness* as it lay for months near death. The point is, animals are *sensitive* to very limited aspects of their environment, and so are we. So we must keep in mind that as we describe our senses, our means of detection, we are dealing with very limited *instruments*.

We are aware of only a very small part of our *surroundings*. (But we can be sure that this is the part that has been important to our survival.) The second problem in describing the senses is that *sensory abilities* may differ widely from one individual to the next. This area is rife with *anecdotes* and untested claims, but there are many substantiated cases of remarkable and unusual keenness of vision, hearing, touch, and so on. What are we to make of people who apparently can "*feel*" the colour beneath their fingers? Of the *ability* of twins in different rooms to silently *communicate*? Of people who can read newspapers across the room or see the moons on other planets?

Here, we're *dangerously* close to leaving the realm of *acceptable* scientific topics and, of course, above all things, we want to be acceptable. So let's just admit that we are aware of only a small part of our environment, and that there may be great differences in the sensory abilities of people, and move on to consider some of the basic mechanisms of perception. We will review only a few basic types of *receptors*, those neural structures that are capable of responding to environmental stimuli, in a few representative groups of animals.

THERMORECEPTORS

Thermoreception is the ability to sense heat. Such an ability is important because the delicate chemical processes of life can normally be *conducted* only within certain *temperature* ranges. A heat-sensitive animal is able to adjust itself in its environment so as to position itself within those ranges.

Not much is known about heat detection in *invertebrates*, and it is assumed that most of them lack *thermoreceptors*. Some, however, do have these sensors. For example, cockroaches have heat *receptors* on their legs, with which they can locate optimal places to live, like your house.

In addition, sensitivity to temperature may be important in helping *parasites* locate their warm-blooded hosts. The *mechanisms* of heat detection in vertebrates are better understood. Some *species*, such as the pit vipers, have been intensively studied, and we have been able to determine how they locate prey by heat detection.

In many *mammals*, including humans, temperature is registered by warm receptors, cold receptors and pain receptors (which register the extremes of temperature). Interestingly, the receptors stop responding when the temperature is constant, but remain responsive if the temperature changes. Thus, standing in a shower that is turning cold is much more startling than standing in a cold shower. Thermal receptors quickly adapt to too cold or too hot so that the temperature becomes bearable.

Thermal receptors are not uniformly distributed over the body. For example, the face and hands are not very sensitive to temperature changes, while the lips and mouth are extremely sensitive.

TACTILE RECEPTORS

Tactile receptors respond to touch. They fire whenever their shape is altered or *distorted*, and they *trigger* extremely sensitive, fast-firing

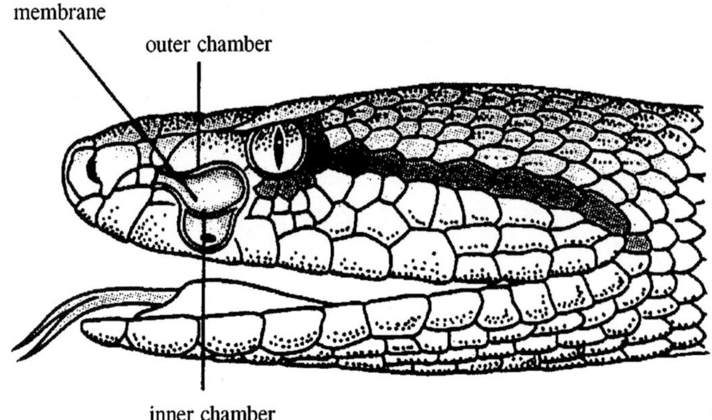

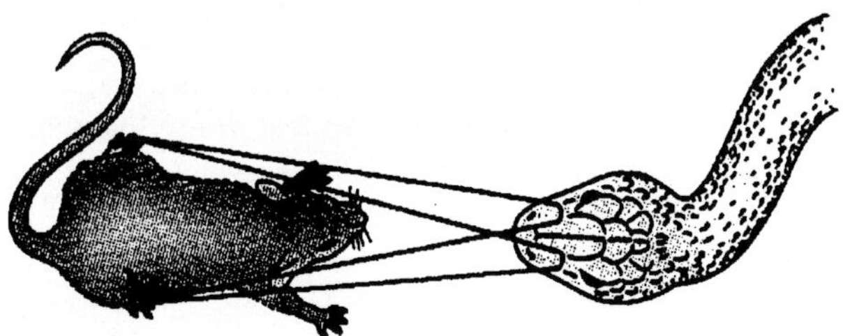

Figure 8.1 : Heat sensors in the pit viper (rattlesnake, crotalus viridis). Pit vipers detect their prey through a pair of heat-sensing deveices located in the deptressions near the eyes.

neurons. In some cases, *bristles*, *whiskers*, or hairs extend from the tissues around these receptors so that objects are perceived by these feelers before they contact living tissue.

Many *invertebrates* have such sensory feelers, as we see in *jumping* spiders. *Web-building* spiders have hairy legs that react to vibrations set up by trapped insects. Tiny hairs on the abdomen of cockroaches are extremely sensitive to light air-currents-such as those produced by a *descending* human foot. Many invertebrates use touch in finding food and mates and in avoiding *predators*.

Vertebrates have two kinds of tactile receptors, those that register pressure and those that respond to touch. The pressure receptors are located deeper under the skin. They are essentially encapsulated nerve endings called *Pacinian corpuscles*. Near the surface of the skin are *Meissner's corpuscles*, which are believed to respond to light touch.

In mammals, certain parts of the body are especially sensitive to touch. A sleeping dog can immediately be aroused if you ouch the hairy area just under its tail (preferably with a stick). In human the most sensitive parts include the *hairy areas* and the genitals, as you have noticed. In all *primates*, most sensitive areas also include the *lips*, the area around the eyes, and uncalloused fingertips. (Can you see the adaptive advantages to *heightened* sensitivity in these areas?)

AUDITORY RECEPTORS

Audition, or hearing, involves the detection of sound, usually a distant stimulus. Most invertebrates lack specific receptors for detecting the vibrating molecules of air that produce sound. However, many are sensitive to the vibration of the air, water, or soil in which they live.

Insects are an exception among the animals without backbones in that some of them can hear quite well. Some, such as grasshoppers and crickets, have *tympanal membranes* that respond to sound much as does the *human eardrum*. One of the best stories regarding the evolution of hearing in insects involves that of noctuid moths.

In general, the hearing structures of land vertebrates include an *auditory canal* and a *tympanic membrane* (ear drum) that vibrates from one to three moveable middle ear bones. The vibrations of the bones then stimulate receptors that carry impulses to the hearing centers of the brain.

The auditory apparatus of mammals is somewhat distinct among the vertebrates. For one thing, most mammals have an *external ear*. This includes the *pinna* and the *auditory canal*. The pinna is the part that can be moved, as we see when a dog focuses on some sound. (Humans have largely lost the ability to move their ears, but those who can manage it are in great demand at social events.)

The auditory canal channels sound toward the *eardrum*, which vibrates in *synchrony* with the *soundwaves*. The vibrating eardrum causes the bones of the middle ear to vibrate. Whereas most other vertebrates have only one bone in the middle ear, mammals have three: the so-called hammer (*malleus*), anvil (*incus*), and stirrup (*stapes*).

Sound vibrations move the hammer, which is pressed against the vibrating eardrum. The movement is transferred to the anvil which then vibrates the stirrup. The stirrup vibrates against the inner ear's *oval window*, which, in turn, sets up movements of the fluid inside the long, coiled *cochlea*.

The cochlea is divided along its length into three long chambers. The base of the central chamber forms the *basilar membrane* from which arise modified cilia ("*hair cells*"). The sound *vibrations* move the

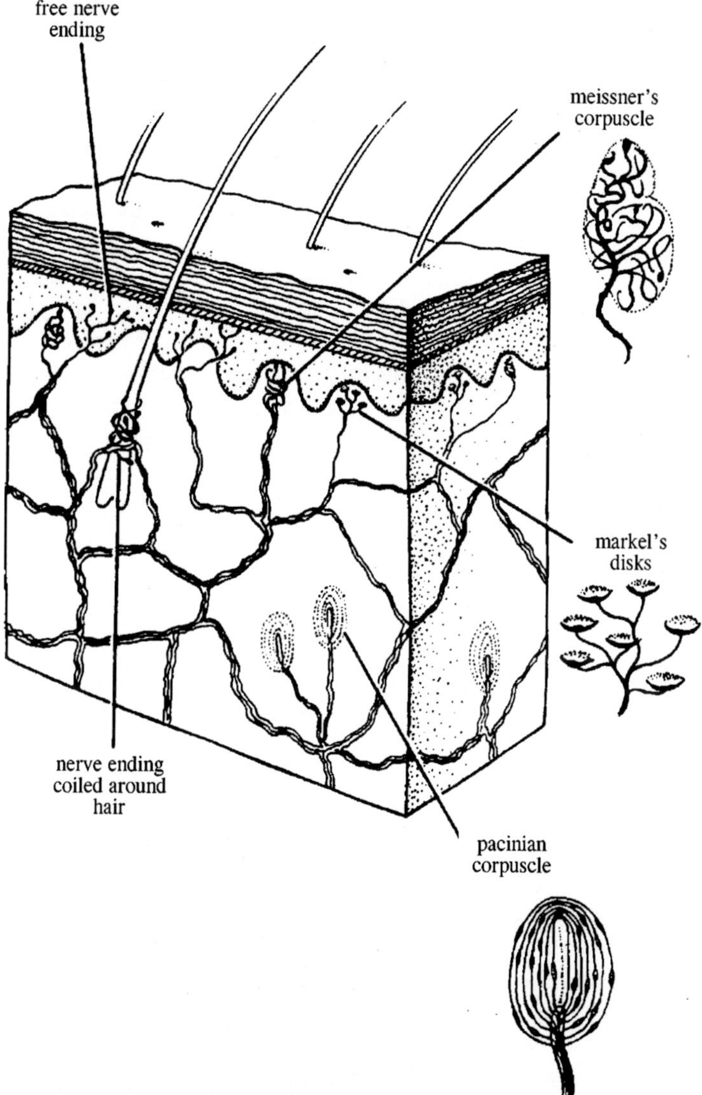

Figure 8.2 : Specialised touch receptors in the skin of human. Meissner's corpuscles are located close to the surface and register light touch.

fluid in the upper chamber of the cochlea, which then presses against the fluid in the middle chamber and moves the basilar membrane.

The hair cells extending from it are attached to a more flexible membrane above, the *tectorial membrane*. As the tectorial membrane moves, impulses directly over the auditory neurons that lead to th brain. Some hearing *impairment* is directly related to the loss of the hair cells, and they can be lost by exposure to loud noise, such as amplified rock music. (In fact, partial loss of hearing is considered a badge of honor among some rock *musicians* and their fans. Others associated with the business are *alarmed* by the trend).

The *basilar* membrane itself is narrower and more rigid near the eardrum, becoming much wider and thinner further away. The pitch of a sound is registered according to which hairs are *stimulated*. High pitches stimulate hairs in the *narrower* regions of the basilar membrane near the oval window; low pitches register at the wider tip of the *coiled* tube, the part lying in the innermost part of the snail-like coil.

Loudness is apparently detected by the number of neurons stimulated and the frequency with which an impulse is generated in each of these neurons. Table elsewhere in this chpater summarises the structure and function of the human ear.

CHEMORECEPTORS

The ability to detect the presence of chemicals is called *chemoreception*, and it varies widely in sensitivity throughout the animal world. If you encounter a *smelly dog*, you should keep in mind that your opinion of his odour pales before his perception of you. We can assume that either dogs don't mind our scent or they're just being *polite*.

Chemoreception involves both *olfaction* (smell) and *gustation* (taste). The mechanisms are essentially similar, but olfaction usually involves distant *stimuli* and *gustation* registers those in which the source is in contact with the receptors.

The most remarkable *chemoreceptive* abilities are found among the insects. In this group, there are taste receptors on various parts of the body, including *mouthparts*, *antennae*, and *forelegs* (since some are known to eat what they walk on). Some can even taste with their *egglaying* organs, an ability that enables them to lay eggs only on certain kinds of plants.

Generally, however, most insect olfactory receptors lie at the ends of minute *tubules* that branch throughout the insect body. *Molecules* that diffuse into a tubule become dissolved in the insect's body fluids and can

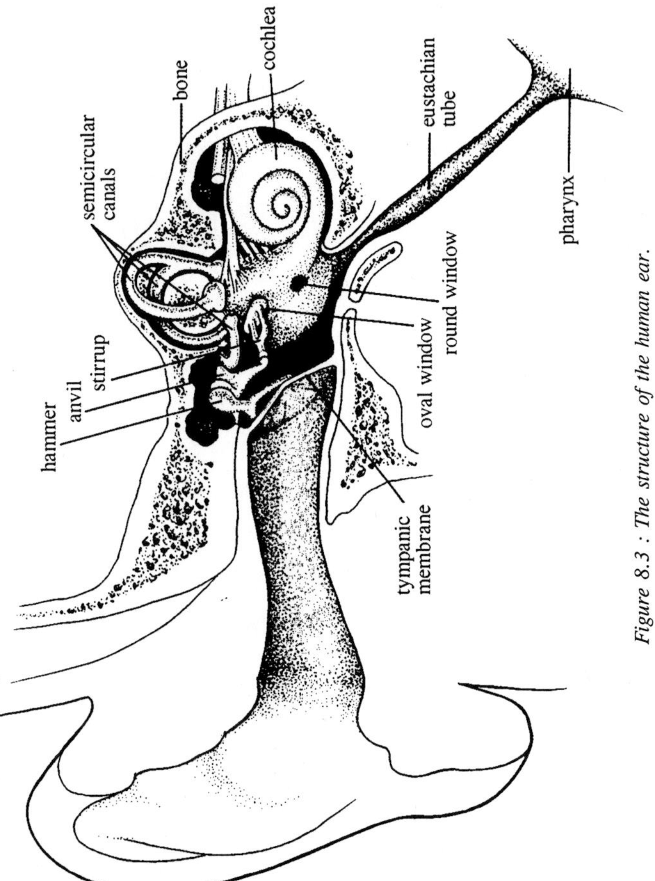

Figure 8.3 : The structure of the human ear.

bind to receptors on the membranes of the tiny sensory cells. (One of the most amazing olfactory abilities is found in the Atlas moth).

Chemoreception in vertebrates usually involves moving chemicals into specialised sacs or tubes that are lined with receptors. The chemicals (as is almost always the case in cellular organisms) must first be dissolved in fluid before they can cross the membranes of the receptors, so these *sacs* and *tubes* are usually moist.

Among vertebrates, mammals have the best sense of smell, with the best smellers being the carnivores and *rodents*. However, some mammals, such as the toothed whales, have no sense of smell at all. The sense of smell is also rather poorly developed in us primates. Chimpanzees, for example, smell about like you do (*no offense*). In

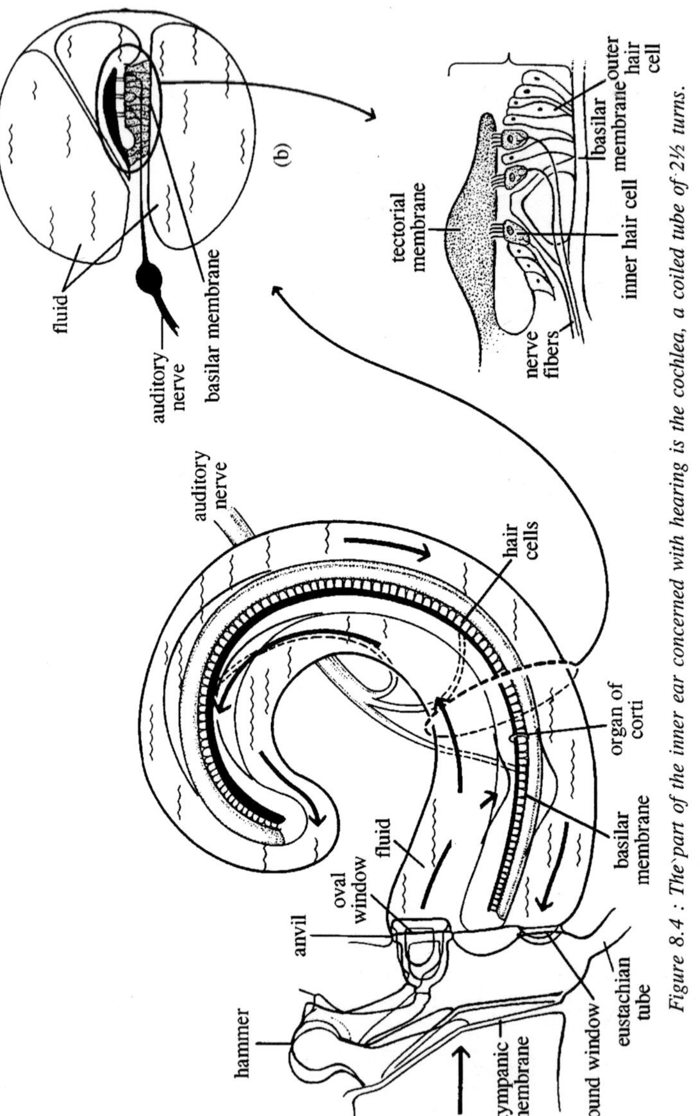

Figure 8.4 : The part of the inner ear concerned with hearing is the cochlea, a coiled tube of 2½ turns.

humans, the olfactory receptors in the nasal passage are connected directly to a slender, forward extension of the brain, called the *olfactory bulb*. Refer back to Figure elsewhere in this chapter and compare the relative sizes of the olfactory bulb in various animals. (It is most reduced in humans-and largest in what group?)

The receptors involved in taste are neurologically very similar to those of smell. It is generally acknowledged that there are four basic tastes: *sweet*, *sour*, *salty*, and *bitter*. In humans, these are located in specific areas of the tongue. Salt can be tasted over the entire surface of the tongue, but sweet registers on the tip, sour on the sides, and bitter on the back.

Research indicates that most cells can respond to three or four tastes, but those of each group are particularly sensitive to a single taste. One might wonder, if a taste receptor can be activated by more than one kind of molecule, how does the *brain respond* properly to each taste? It turns out that each kind of chemical produces a distinctive pattern of neural firing in the *receptors*, and the brain deciphers each pattern.

The tasting abilities of some individuals is highly developed, due

Table 8.1 : Structure of the Ear.

Structure	*Description*	*Function*
External Ear		
pinna	part of ear outside the head	catch and direct sound
auditory canal	tube between pinna and eardrum	channel sound to middle ear
Middle Ear		
tympanic membrane (eardrum)	vibratory membrane	vibrates in response to sound
hammer (malleus) anvil (incus) stapes (stirrup)	three small bones in middle ear	transmit vibrations of eardrum to inner ear; increase force of vibration
Inner Ear		
sacs and semicircular canals	two fluid-filled chambers and three bony canals at right angles to one another	equilibrium
cochlea	fluid-filled snail-shaped bone, containing hair cells; auditory nerve starts here	houses organ of hearing which generates nerve impulses

to either heightened sensitivity of receptors or a *well-trained* ability to recognise certain tastes. Wine tasters are among the most highly trained *chemodetectors*. Chemoreception has been extremely important in the evolutionary history of humans. In essence, it gives us information about the environment before we are forced to interact with it.

It lets us know what is good and desirable as well as those things that are to be avoided. For example, sweet is the taste of carbohydrates (ripe fruit tastes sweet). *Unripe* fruit, however, may be sour, and we have little tolerance for that taste. This means that we are not likely to eat unripe fruit but will probably wait until it has *matured* and its food value is higher.

Bitter, we might mention, is the taste of a number of powerful poisons and can *trigger* a *gag reflex* at the back of the tongue. We probably have a great deal to learn about the role of chemoreception in human life. For example, recent research has focused on the role of smell in sexual attractiveness.

There is evidence that masking *human odour* with *colognes* might be counterproductive in increasing one's appeal. It has been suggested that the hair on some part of our bodies may be useful in trapping our odours and aiding in subtle communication with the opposite sex. (One might think that the communication had best be very *subtle*).

In addition, preliminary experiments show that people can generally distinguish between males and females on the basis of both breath and body scent. The *groundwork* has been laid for what should be some *fascinating* lines of research.

PROPRIOCEPTORS

Proprioceptors sense the position of various parts of the body. They tell you where your body parts are relative to one another. (That seems a good thing to know.) This is an area that perhaps has not received enough research attention, but that may be because it normally works so efficiently.

Proprioception is common in many invertebrates and is achieved by receptors that respond to *pressure*, *stretching*, and *bending*. In some insects these sensors are at the base of hairs, while in crustaceans, such as lobsters, the receptors are within the muscles. Among *vertebrates*, certain kinds of *proprioceptors* are also concentrated deep within the muscles.

They are stimulated as the muscle *stretches* and places pressure on them. It is apparent that proprioception is particularly important among

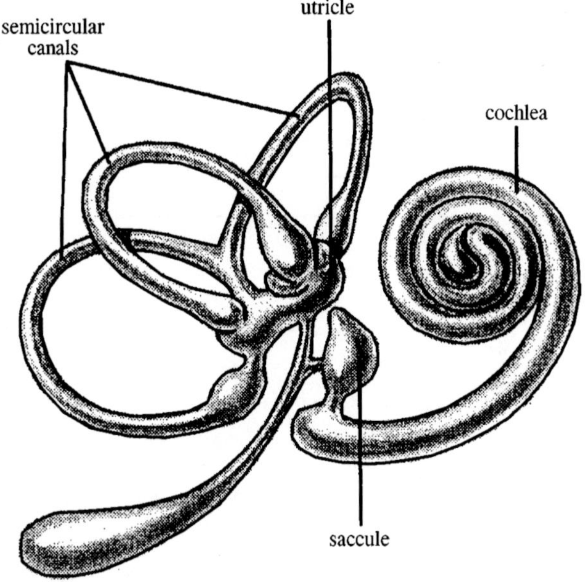

Figure 8.5 : Semicircular canals.

the more active or athletic vertebrates. Clumsy monkeys would tend to fall out of trees, and so we find that monkeys have, in fact, many proprioceptors.

Vertebrates also have very precise equilibrium proprioceptors located in the inner ear. In most species, there are three fluid-filled loops, or *semi-circular canals*, opening to two chambers. Each canal is filled with fluid and contains sensory hairs. Any change in the animal's position results in movement of the fluid, which then stimulates the hairs.

Since the canals lie at right angles to each other, movement in any direction can be detected. The chambers are called the *utricle* and *saccule*, and they contain small granules that shift when the body moves, stimulating the sensory hairs and providing information on the position of the head with respect to *gravity*.

VISUAL RECEPTORS

Humans are highly visual animals, and so we have a keen interest in sight. However, compared to some animals, especially birds, we don't see well at all. There is indeed a great deal of variation in visual ability among animals, and, not *surprisingly*, the ability is correlated with a *species'* simple need to see.

But how exactly is any visual receptor stimulated? And what

stimulates it? In essence, it is sensitive to a particular part of the electromagnetic spectrum we call light. Light's wavelength ranges from about 430 nm (nanometers) to 750 nm, but no animal can see more than part of this range.

Table 8.2 : Structure of the Eye.

Structure	***Description***	***Function***
Pupil	open center of iris	entrance for incoming light
Iris	the coloured, part of eye	regulates the amount of light that enters eye
Cornea	transparent dome of tissue at front of eye	bends light rays to help focus them on retina
Lens	semi-spherical transparent body of tissue	adjustable focusing of light rays onto photoreceptors
Aqueous humor	clear fluid between tens and cornea	transmits and bends light; pressure of fluid helps maintain shape of eye
Vitreous humor	jellylike substance within chamber behind lens	transmits and bends light; pressure of substance helps maintain shape of eye
Retina	tissue containing rods and cones	sensory area; receives light and generates nerve impulses
Fovea	tiny pit on retina with a high density of cones	most sensitive part of retina
Optic nerve	bundle of nerve fibers leaving eye	carries signals from retina to brain

The shorter wavelengths, such as x-rays, beta rays, and *gamma* rays can't be detected by any animals, nor can the very long ones, such as radio waves. The detectable waves are absorbed by special *visual pigments* that then transform the wave energy into a neural stimulus.

In vertebrates, the light-sensitive part of the eye is the *retina*. It is composed of two kinds of cells, *rods* (specialised to detect light) and *cones* (specialised for colour). The rods hold large amounts of a pigment called *visual purple*. When this pigment is activated by light, it "bleaches" and the permeability of the rod changes. The change in permeability causes electrochemical changes that may lead to action potentials (impulses) that will be sent to the brain where they will be deciphered and integrated.

Whereas rods are sensitive to all wavelengths of visible light, cones respond only to specific wavelengths-that is, to specific colours. Humans and other primates have three kinds of cones that respond either to red, green, or blue. The *multitude* of colours we see depends on the *interplay* between these three.

The real question is, of course, do bulls see red? The answer is, not very well, if at all. (Cats may be able to barely detect red, but they cannot be *depended* upon to charge red capes.) In fact, real colour vision is found only among some species of insects, fishes, reptiles, and birds, and among *mammals*. (In this last group, the primates are the colour specialists.)

Since life is an *opportunistic phenomenon*, living things must have ways of detecting their opportunities (and minimising their risks). This detection, we see, is the result of a *dazzling* interplay among a host of specialised receptors that comprise the senses. Next we will see just how animals use this information to get along in their special parts of the *world*.

9

Nerves and Hormones

Most people living in the nineteenth century never thought to explain life in chemical and physical terms. Without understanding enzymes, metabolic pathways, or the basis of inheritance, even the best-educated individuals could find cells incomprehensible. Did not organisms operate by processes that were impossible to duplicate outside cells? And wasn't it likely that these processes depended on an inherited "*vital spirit*" that traced ultimately to a supernatural Creator?

Not all nineteenth-century biologists subscribed to this concept of *vitalism*. Other scientists believed that if only they knew enough specific details, organisms could be explained in *mechanistic* terms. Over the past hundred years chemical investigations have revealed so much about cells, and so many cellular processes have been carried out in the test tube that for most scientists the vitalism-mechanism argument is dead.

Of course, no one has created a cell, but we believe this fact is due to the complexity of cells, not to the fundamental nature of their processes. Having grown up in the twentieth century, you probably find mechanistic explanations easy to accept, at least for some processes. We have shown that digestion is a chemical and physical process. Similarly, you understand why energy is necessary to sustain life.

You also know that we acquire energy in our food, and you can trace the metabolic processes that convert food energy into ATP energy. Despite this ready acceptance of mechanistic explanations of certain basic body processes, do you associate your personal experiences with atoms?

Does it seem plausible that pain, pleasure, memory, reasoning, and even love result from molecules and their behaviour?

Although we don't have the details or even a good outline of all the processes in the nervous system, we believe that the poetry of Homer, the concertos of Rachmaninoff, and the dreams of Martin Luther King, Jr., involved the spin of electrons.

So do the notes you take in history class, the indecision you feel facing a yellow light, and everything else you create or experience. To maintain homeostasis, most animals depend on two interrelated systems. The *nervous* system integrates information about internal and external conditions and coordinates responses through cell-to-cell stimulation.

The *endocrine system* also responds to internal conditions and coordinates responses, but through cell secretions that are carried in body fluids. In animals such as ourselves most of these messengers are carried in the blood; we call them *hormones*. Hormones are so important that we have mentioned several in earlier discussions of body activities.' In the latter part of the present chapter, we will emphasize the similarities between endocrine cells and nerve cells and show that the endocrine system is largely controlled by the nervous system.

NEURAL COORDINATION

The nervous system of vertebrates is tremendously complex. It extends throughout the body and is composed of billions of cells. Many of these cells are *neurons* (nerve cells). Other cells of the nervous system support and nourish neurons and, perhaps, have other yet-to-be-explained duties.

Because the nervous system fans so widely through the body and is so intricate, any classification of the parts must be an oversimplification. But for convenience we speak of the brain and spinal cord as the *central nervous system*.

The brain, of course, is a massive structure within the skull cavity. The spinal cord extends from the skull and passes through channels in the vertebral column (backbones). Nerves and associated structures that extend from the brain or spinal cord into the remainder of the body constitute the *peripheral nervous system*. But the central and peripheral nervous systems are no more separate than are your heart and blood vessels. In fact, many neurons extend within both "*systems*".

You will also read about the *autonomic nervous system*, a term that is engrained in the vocabulary of both biologists and psychologists. It is unfortunate that this term has become so established, because the "*autonomic nervous system*" not only is part of the nervous system but actually includes portions of both the "central" and "peripheral" nervous systems.

You see, autonomic nervous system is a term for those neural structures that control internal organs. (The term "*autonomic*" refers to the seemingly automatic nature of this action that ordinarily occurs beyond our conscious control.) Rest assured, you have not three nervous systems but really only one.

Neurons and Neural Organisation

Nerve cells are highly specialised. Each consists of a large "cell body" and one or more "*nerve fibers.*" The *cell body* of a neuron contains the nucleus and the usual cytoplasmic structures. The *nerve fibers* are extensions, often extremely long, of the cytoplasm. In humans some of the longest nerve fibers extend from the spinal cord at shoulder level clear to the tips of the fingers.

Others reach from the lower back to the toes. Most neurons bear some nerve fibers that are *dendrites*. These are highly branched and often knobby. Dendrites receive incoming signals and transmit them toward the cell body.

Usually one fiber, the *axon*, carries messages away from the cell body. At a *synapse*, the region where two neurons meet, it is the axon of one neuron that passes the message to a dendrite of the second neuron. Axons are of uniform diameter throughout and usually branch only toward the end. Long nerve fibers are generally covered with *myelin sheaths*, which are actually portions of surrounding cells wrapped around the nerve fiber.

The sheath cells are drawn so thin and wrapped so tightly that the myelin sheath is little more than the plasma membranes of the sheathing cells. The high lipid content of these cell membranes gives myelin sheaths a whitish, greasy appearance.

Not only are many neurons fantastically long and structurally specialised; they are also unusually active metabolically. Neurons use a great deal of energy and are extremely busy at protein synthesis. These expenditures maintain highly organised structural and chemical systems that permit the neuron to transmit impulses.

Neurons are classified according to their functions. *Sensory neurons* are those of the peripheral nervous system that transmit impulses from sense organs to the central nervous system. *Motor neurons* deliver messages from the brain or spinal cord through the peripheral nervous

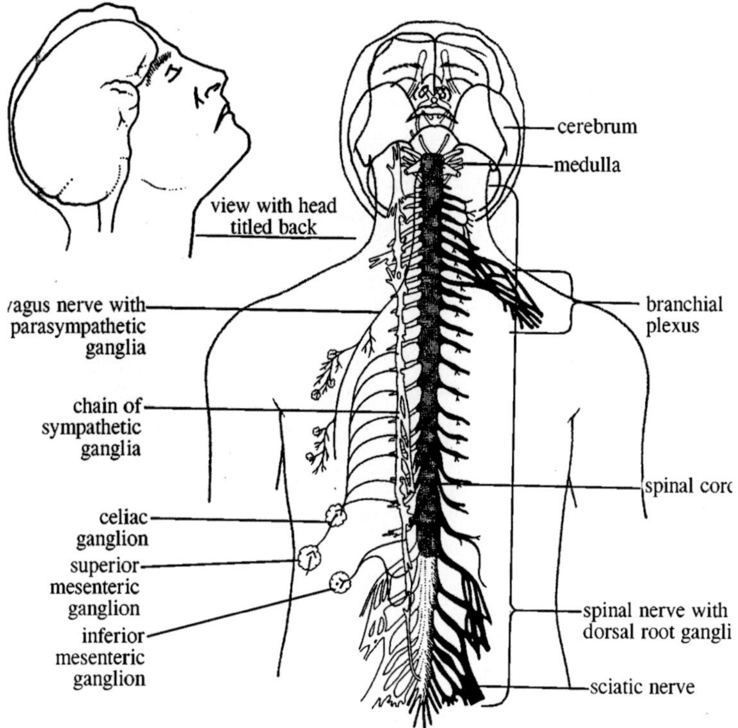

Figure 9.1. The Human Nervous System.

system to individual muscles and glands. Actually these activities are only a tiny part of the work of neurons. Most neurons are involved in storage of information, correlation of new information with old information, and decisions about responses. We lump these functions together as *integration*. The cells that carry out integration are called *interneurons*. Such interneurons compose over 90 percent of the mass of the central nervous system.

Nerves versus Neurons

Don't confuse nerves with neurons. Nerves are bundles of nerve fibers from many different neurons. A large nerve may consist of hundreds of fibers, both axons and dendrites. They are held together by sturdy coats of connective tissue supplied with numerous small blood vessels.

The cell bodies of most neurons, including many with fibers that lie in nerves, are located in the brain or spinal cord. However, the neurons of the sensory nerves are one exception. The cell bodies of

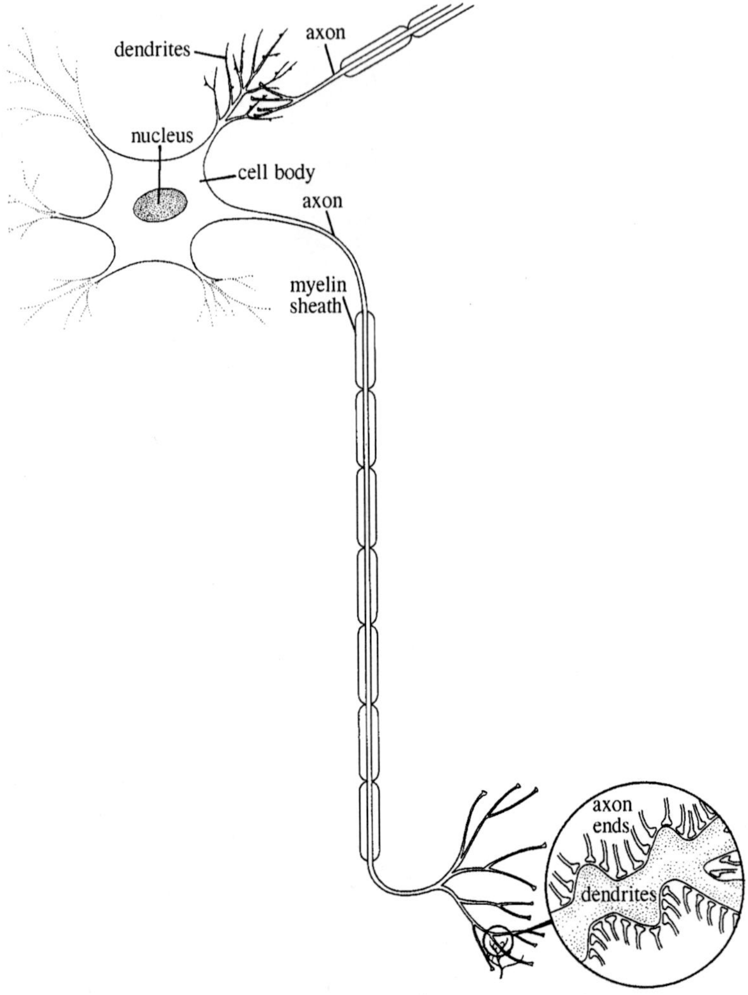

Figure 9.2 : Neurons.

these neurons lie together in clumps at the base of the spinal nerves. Any such clump of cell bodies on a peripheral nerve is known as a *ganglion*. Other ganglia include those of the autonomic nervous system.

The Central Nervous System

The arrangement of neurons determines the organisation of the brain and spinal cord. Although these two structures are continuous and similar in many ways, the spinal cord is definitely simpler.

A cross section through the spinal cord reveals a butterfly-shaped

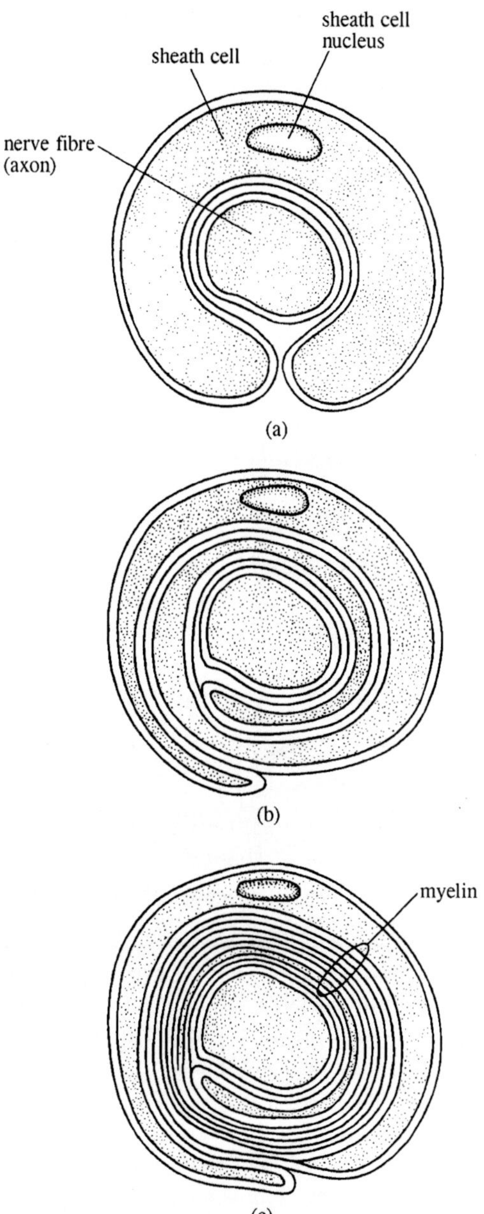

Figure 9.3 : "Myelin Sheath" The sheath that covers most long nerve fibers consists largely of many layers of plasma membranes belonging to sheath cells.

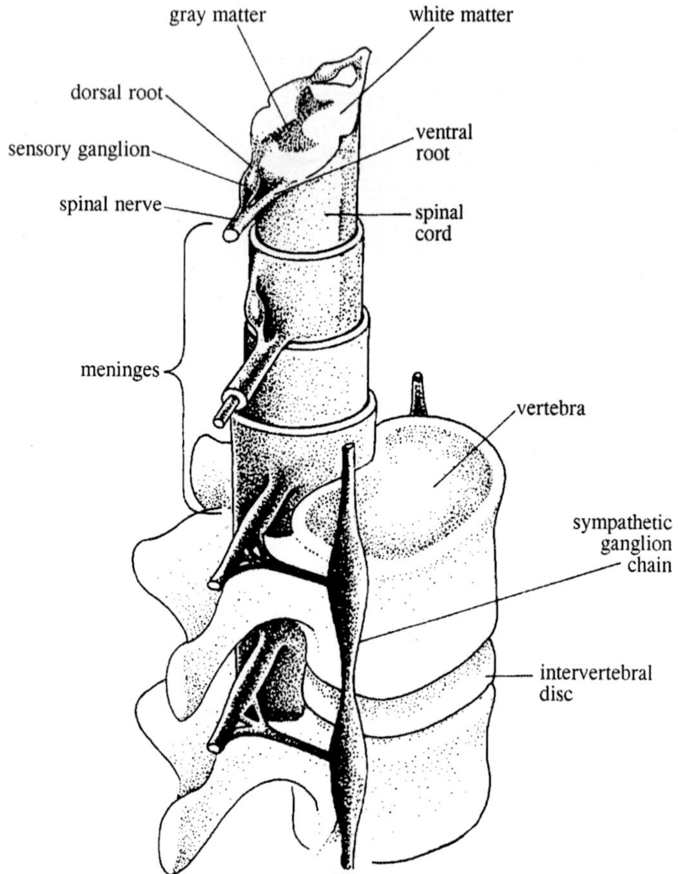

Figure 9.4 : "Spinal Cord" Three connective-tissue layers, known as the meninges, enclose the spinal cord, which is further protected by the vertebrae through which it passes. Because the spinal cord lies within the bony vertebral column, the spinal nerves must emerge between the vertebrae.

core of "gray matter" embedded in glistening "white matter." *White matter* consists of tracts of myelinated fibers that carry information up or down the cord. Through the white matter, messages pass from the cord to the brain and vice versa.

Messages also pass from one level of the cord to another. *Gray matter*, on the other hand, consists of masses of cells bodies, as well as unmyelinated fibers. Because there is no myelin sheathing, this tissue has a grayish cast. Synapses occur in gray matter but not in white matter. Just as the nerves are wrapped in connective tissue and supplied with blood vessels, so are the brain and spinal cord. Between the central nervous system and the bones of the skull and vertebral column, there lie a series of membranes, the *meninges*.

The outer layer is especially tough. The inner two layers are separated by a lymphlike fluid that cushions the nervous system against physical blows. Because this *cerebrospinal fluid* originates within the brain and is in communication with brain tissues, its composition can provide clues to conditions deep inside.

Infections, hemorrhages, and many diseases alter the cerebrospinal fluid. Liquid for diagnosis can be withdrawn harmlessly. Physicians use a long needle to tap a reservoir of cerebrospinal fluid in the meninges near the base of the spinal cord.

NERVE IMPULSES

The characteristic activity of neurons is the transmission of messages, or *impulses*, as they are called, from one to another. The ability of cells to transmit impulses arises from the unequal distribution of ions' on either side of the plasma membrane. And since ions are electrically charged, the unequal distribution produces an electrical potential across the membrane.

One can measure it by placing a tiny electrode inside a neuron and another outside, then connecting the two through a voltmeter. The *resting potential* of a neuron (that is, the potential of one not sending an impulse) is about 70 millivolts, or 70/1000 of a volt. The inside of the neuron is negative with respect to the outside.

Chemically, the positive ions are mainly sodium and potassium, whereas the negative ions that are concentrated on the inside include large organic substances, such as amino acids, proteins, and nucleic acids. There is a high concentration of sodium ions (Na^+) outside the cell and a substantial concentration of potassium (K^+) inside. This unequal distribution is maintained by a *sodium-potassium pump*, an

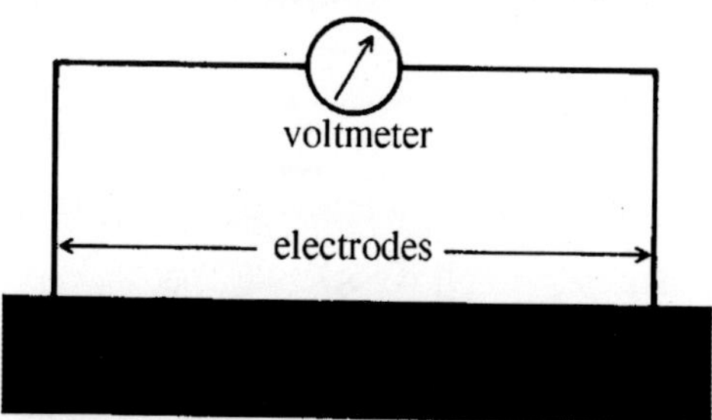

Figure 9.5 : Apparatus for measurement of electrical potential in Nerve Fibers.

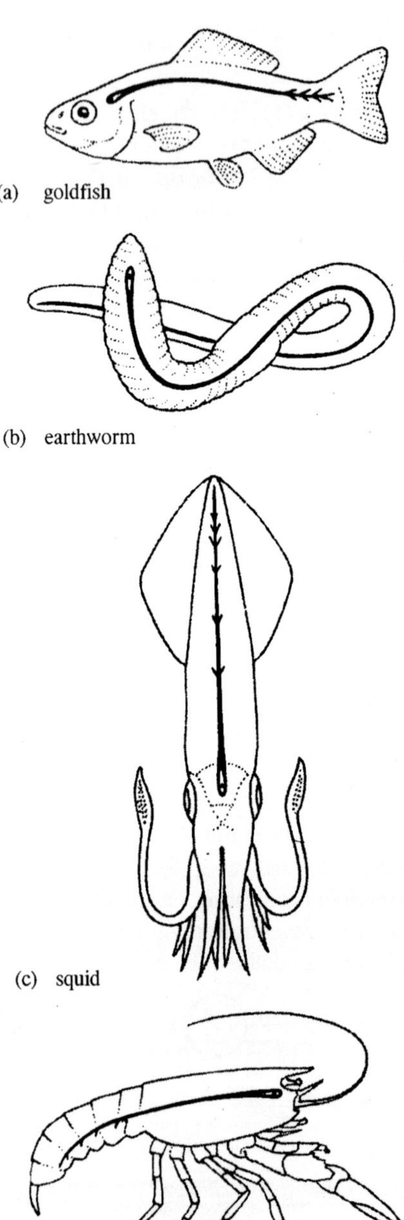

Figure 9.6 : Giant Neurons.

activetransport system that pumps sodium out of cells and potassium into cells.

In this process energy is used to collect sodium ions from inside the cell, where they are scarce, and move them to the outside where sodium is more abundant. At the same time that the pump is exchanging sodium ions for potassium ions and thereby concentrating potassium inside the cell, the small size of potassium ions permits them to leak out.

This outward diffusion of positively charged potassium ions and the fact that large negatively charged organic ions are trapped inside the membrane results in more negative ions inside than outside. The resulting difference in electrical charges is the source of the resting potential.

Action Potential

Neurons respond to a variety of stimuli that temporarily inactivate the sodium-potassium pump. Such stimulation alters the distribution of sodium and potassium ions. When the pump is inactivated, sodium ions flood into the nerve cell. As more and more positively charged sodiums diffuse into the neuron, its electrical potential begins to drop, and the cell membrane becomes depolarised.

At this point there is no charge difference between the inside and the outside. Then, for a fraction of a second as sodium ions continue to flood into the neuron, the inside of the cell actually becomes positive, relative to the outside. This *action potential* persists for only a few milliseconds before the membrane recovers and restores the resting potential.

Depolarization does not occur over the entire neural membrane at once. Instead, a wave of depolarization sweeps over the neuron from the point of stimulation. Depolarization at one point triggers the depolarization of adjacent regions of the membrane. In other words, depolarization is self-propagating.

The process spreads along the entire length of the neuron, constituting a *nerve impulse*. After experiencing one wave of depolarization, a neuron cannot respond to a second stimulation until the sodium-potassium pump reestablishes the original distribution of ions.

All or Nothing

Neurons do not send an impulse in response to just any stimulus. Only stimuli of a certain minimum strength, or *threshhold value*, can cause an impulse to be propagated. A minor stimulus may produce a partial depolarization of the membrane, but such a depolarization will spread only a short distance and then die out. However, once a depolarization of sufficient magnitude is established, a nerve impulse is inevitable.

A nerve impulse is an *all-or-none phenomenon*, just as is firing a gun. You can slowly increase pressure on a gun trigger with no effect-up to a point. Once the pressure is sufficient to cause the hammer to strike the cartridge and explode the powder, the bullet inevitably shoots forth.

We all know that we can distinguish between different intensities of stimulation. How can we reconcile this with the all-or-none nature of nerve impulses? The answer is that increases in intensity of stimulation of sense receptors are reflected in increased frequency of impulses in sensory neurons. from these organs.

The greater the intensity of the stimulus, the more times the neurons fire. A strong stimulation sends a series of impulses down the neurons, one after the other. In addition, neurons differ in their sensitivity to stimuli. A mild stimulus to a sense organ will result in depolarization of only some of the neurons serving this organ. A stronger stimulus will recruit the response of a larger number of cells.

Not a Current

Although we have discussed nerve impulses in electrical terms, it would be a grave mistake to assume that the nerve impulse that passes along a fiber is an electrical current. Two observations may help you remember this critical distinction. First, a nerve impulse is due to the movement of ions, not electrons, as in electricity. This movement of ions occurs *across* the membrane depolarizing it.

The impulse that moves along the fiber is a movement in the location where depolarization is occurring at any given moment. Second, an electric current such as operates an electric toaster moves three million times faster than does a nerve impulse. Electricity travels at the speed of light (299,800 kilometers or 186,000 miles per second). Messages from your brain to your toe move no more than 100 meters (325 feet) per second.

From One Neuron to Another

Usually a nerve impulse must move from one neuron to another in order to reach its final destination. Neurons form distinct patterns; the axonic end of one neuron branches and abuts on the dendritic ends of several other neurons. But adjacent nerve fibers never actually touch. There is a very narrow gap at each *synapse*, or junction. The manner in which nerve impulses bridge the synaptic gap has important consequences.

Once initiated, a nerve impulse is transmitted along the surface of a neuron in all directions from the site of stimulus. But the impulse does not pass randomly to all connecting neurons. If it did, any stimulus would provoke a generalised response throughout the body. Instead, nerve impulses can be transmitted across a synapse in only one direction. For this reason, our responses to stimuli can be highly specific actions. The one-way nature of synapses results from differences in the two sides of the synapse.

Nerve impulses can pass only from the axon of one neuron to a dendrite on the next. Close inspection reveals that the tips of axons are swollen. These bulbous ends of axons contain membrane-bound sacs of neurotransmitters. *Neurotransmitters* are chemicals that can alter the permeability of the membrane of dendrites and thus either cause or prevent an impulse in the neuron affected. When a nerve impulse reaches the tip of an axon, it causes the tiny sacs of neurotransmitters to move to the synaptic surface.

Here the sacs burst and release their contents into the gap between the axon and the dendrite. The released chemicals diffuse across the gap, where they alter the membrane of the dendrite.

Neurotransmitters released by axons combine with specific sites on dendrites. Since there are several kinds of neurotransmitters, there are also several kinds of receptors. It is important to recognise that *neurotransmitters are secreted* by axons. Thus there is a fundamental similarity between functions of neurons and of the endocrine tissues that produce hormones. Both secrete chemicals that have specific effects on other cells and that are effective in tiny quantities.

Since neurotransmitters alter dendrite membranes, it is essential that the transmitters be removed so that the dendrite can recover and be ready to respond to subsequent signals. Different neurotransmitters are removed in different ways, but the bestknown transmitter, *acetylcholine*, is destroyed by an enzyme. This enzyme, *cholinesterase*, is normally present in the synapse.

Inhibitors of cholinesterase cause havoc in the nervous system. Nerve gases developed for biological warfare include cholinesterase inhibitors. So do the organophosphate insecticides. Insects seem more susceptible than people to these pesticides, and the small body size of insects makes them more vulnerable to small amounts of the chemical. Nonetheless, these substances are also dangerous to people.

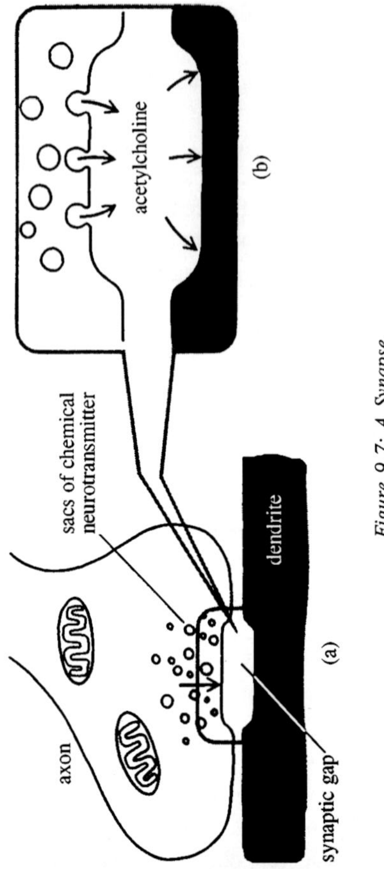

Figure 9.7: A Synapse.

REFLEXES: SMALL SCALE EXAMPLES OF NEURAL FUNCTION

To comprehend how the nervous system works we need to understand how neurons interact. The examples provided by reflexes are easy to analyze and may illustrate processes at work in more complex activity.

A *reflex* is a behaviour pattern that is predictable, adaptive, and automatic. Consider the reflexes that occur when a person steps on a tack. Invariably, the stimulus of the tack causes the injured foot to be withdrawn quickly while the opposite leg is rigidly extended. The adaptive value of these reflex actions is clear.

Withdrawing the damaged foot prevents further injury. Contraction of muscles on both sides of the opposite leg locks the leg straight and makes it a stable support for the body. Reflexes such as these occur

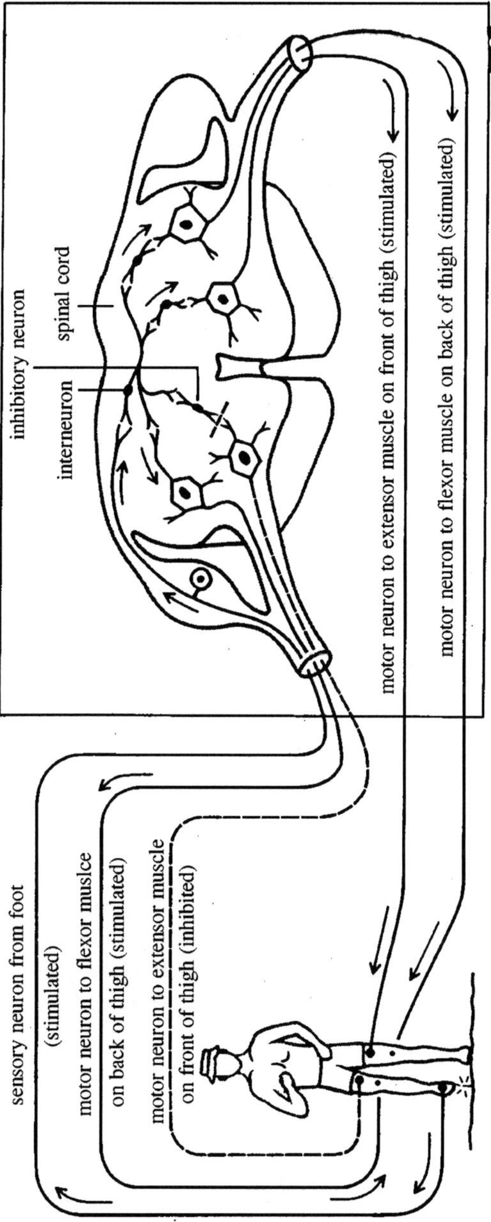

Figure 9.8 : Reflex response to painful stimulus.

without conscious decision and therefore are said to be automatic. Reflexes involve series of components that form reflex arcs.

At a minimum a *reflex arc* includes a sense organ, a sensory neuron, a motor neuron, and an effector, such as a muscle. The *sense organ* receives the stimulus and initiates depolarization of the *sensory neuron*, which passes from the sense organ into the central nervous system.

Within the central nervous system the sensory neuron either synapses directly with a *motor neuron* or indirectly through one or more *interneurons*. The axons of the motor neurons extend to the *muscle or gland* that produces the response.

When you step on a tack, impulses pass from sensory neurons through interneurons to motor neurons that cause the affected leg to bend. Interneurons also carry impulses that cause the opposite leg to be extended. Still other neurons transmit impulses to the brain and permit you to be aware of the tack.

Inhibition

The components outlined above may seem to explain responses to stepping on a tack, but in truth, there is more to the story. These reflexes involve neurons that inhibit as well as those that stimulate. Normally when you stand, the muscles on both the front and back of your legs are partially contracted. Such contraction results from balance reflexes.

If you start to fall forward, the muscles in the back of the leg are stimulated to contract. If you start to fall backward, the muscles in the front of the leg are stimulated to contract. These reflexes are finely tuned so that both sets of muscles contract gently and continuously as you keep your balance.

But consider the effect on these balance reflexes when you step on a tack and another reflex initiates powerful contractions of muscles on the back of the leg. Clearly, the balance reflex would cause the opposing muscles on the front of the leg to contract and prevent the leg from bending.

Withdrawal from the painful tack is possible only if passage of motor impulses to the front muscles is inhibited. Such inhibition is a necessary part of almost all neural activity.

Inhibition occurs at synapses. The dendrites of neurons receive axons from numerous other neurons.

Certain axons release neurotransmitters that make depolarization of the dendritic membrane more difficult. The process may involve increased polarization or other mechanisms. Odd as it may seem, one neurotransmitter can be inhibitory to some cells and stimulatory to others.

Making It Easier

Reflexes also provide examples of facilitation, in which passage of the neural message across the synapse happens more readily. Probably you recognise that your reflexes are more sensitive at some times than at others. We say that we are "nervous" or "jumpy" or "edgy" on days when we respond dramatically to minor stimuli. At other times we are depressed-and so are our reflexes.

These changes in how we feel and behave reflect differences in facilitation impulses that originate in the brain. The differences in facilitation reflect, in turn, the ease with which neurons are depolarized. Stimulation of a neuron by certain axons will facilitate the passage of a nerve impulse from other axons to that neuron.

Perhaps the neurotransmitter substances released by several neurons add together to produce sufficient depolarization to create an action potential. Inhibition and facilitation are major factors in the integration of the nervous system, and they are involved in far more than simple reflexes.

The Brain: Regions and Their Work

As we have indicated, the brain shares a basic organisational pattern with the spinal cord. Both originate from a single embryonic neural tube. In all vertebrates the brain begins as three enlargements on the anterior end of this tube. The spinal cord develops from the remainder.

Each of the three initial swellings form certain important brain regions, and each is also associated with a major sense organ. For a brief description of these regions and their associated sense organs, see Table elsewhere in this chpater.

It would be convenient if we could assign a different function to each brain part, but the truth is that most brain activities require the coordinated action of several regions. The following description is far from complete. We omit many regions and volumes of details concerning functions.

The Most Human Part

The convoluted outer *cortex* of the cerebrum consists of gray matter containing billions of interneurons. These interneurons are involved in

Table 9.1 : Basic Brain Regions and Associated Senses.

Embryonic Regions	*Major Adult Regions*	*Major Senses*
Forebrain	Cerebrum Hypothalamus	Smell
Midbrain	Optic lobes of lower vertebrates In mammals mainly a relay station for vision impulses to the cerebrum, where major sight centers lie	Sight
Hindbrain	Cerebellum Medulla (part of brain stem; connects cerebrum, cerebellum, and spinal cord)	Hearing and balance

reasoning, will power, and other "higher" attributes, as well as control of conscious movement and awareness of sensation. The cerebral cortex is the part of the brain that has changed most during the evolution of mammals. Indeed, the dominant role of the cerebrum is one of the distinguishing features of humans and other primates.

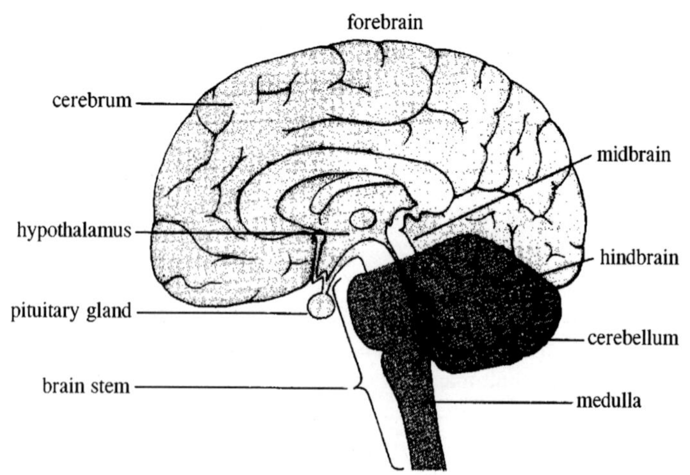

Figure 9.9 : The major brain regions are evident in a section that divides the brain into right and left halves.

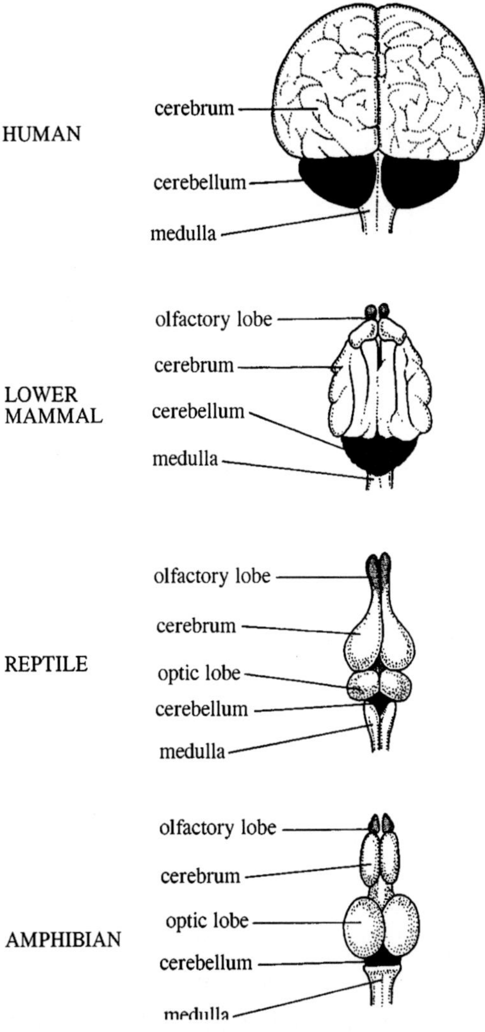

Figure 9.10 : Relative Proportions in Vertebrate Brains.

Stimulation of specific areas in the *motor* region of the cerebral cortex results in movement of specific body parts. This has been known for years, and the motor cortex is thoroughly mapped.

From Figure elsewhere in this chapter it is evident that those body regions possessing the greatest dexterity (such as the lips and fingers) are controlled by areas of the cortex that are relatively larger than those governing regions engaged in only gross movements (e.g.,

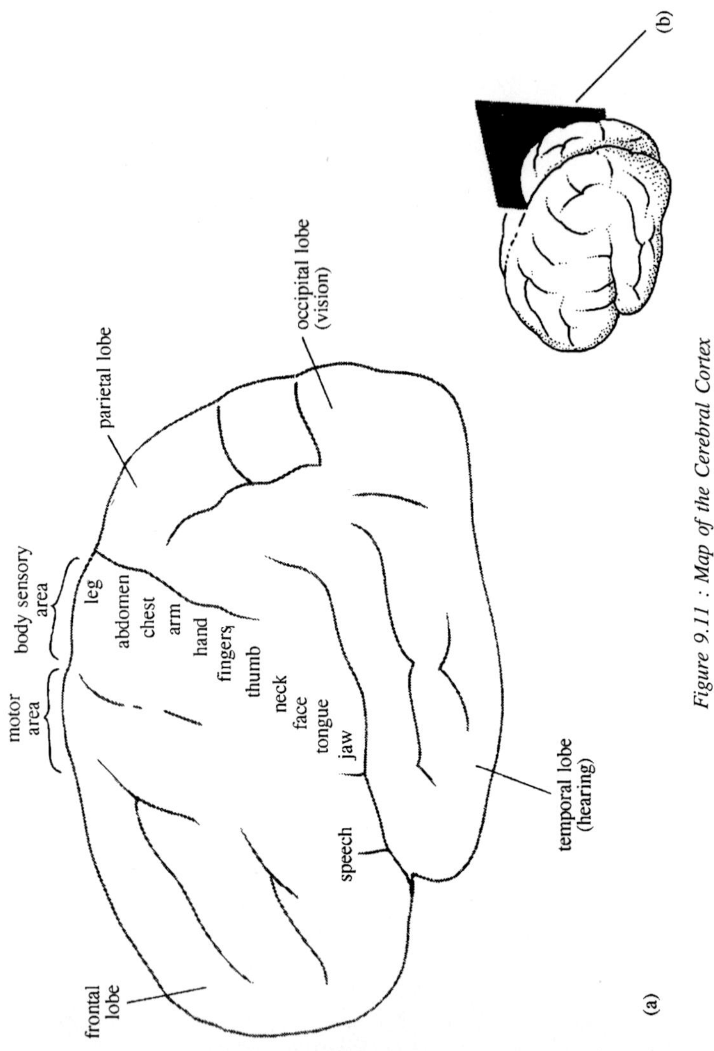

Figure 9.11 : Map of the Cerebral Cortex

the thighs). Whether or not specific cortical neurons control specific muscles remains uncertain.

It is puzzling that mild stimulation of a particular region causes contraction of certain muscles, but that stronger stimulation of other areas causes the same muscles to respond. Furthermore, complete loss of a given portion of the motor cortex does not always result in permanent paralysis of the region of the body it previously controlled.

Posterior to the motor areas lies a *sensory area*. Touch, pressure, temperature, and pain in the skin, muscles, and other body parts seem to be reflected here in a pattern similar to that for the motor regions of the cortex. Tumors and accidental damage to other regions of the cortex produce predictable loss of vision, speech, and hearing. Accordingly, these appear to be localised as shown in Figure elsewhere in this chapter.

A deep furrow separates the cerebrum into right and left hemispheres, and both halves contain many similar areas. Neural pathways from the motor cortex cross from one side of the brain to the other before entering the spinal cord. This is why interruption of the blood supply on one side of the cerebrum (as may happen during a stroke) paralyzes the opposite side of the body.

One-sided Specialisation

Some functions must be localised in only one side of the cortex even if they involve actions of both sides of the body. For example, at any one time there can be only one speech pattern and one will. If any meaning is to be expressed, the two sides of the brain can't act independently. One side must dominate.

Nevertheless, both sides of the cerebrum have the potential for independent action. If the fibers connecting the right and left cerebral hemispheres of the cat are destroyed, each side can learn independently. The two halves can even learn contradictory patterns. In humans, the two halves of the cerebrum are sometimes surgically separated as a treatment for severe epilepsy.

After such operations the individuals seem normal in many ways, but they suffer subtle handicaps. These become evident when patients are dealing with objects they cannot see but can feel. They can call out the name of objects felt with the right hand only but not the names of those felt with the left hand alone. Nevertheless, these individuals do recognise objects touched only with the left hand.

When given number-shaped objects, split-brain humans can signify their recognition by holding up the correct number of fingers. These and other observations on brain-damaged people are consistent with the belief that speech and writing are usually localised in the left cerebrum. (Remember that the left side of the brain connects to the right side of the body, and the right side of the brain connects to the left side of the body.) Spatial interpretation and musical ability reside primarily in the right cerebrum.

The Cerebral Cortex in Motor Activities

Both normal development and severe malformation throw light on how the cerebral cortex dominates motor activities. Newborn babies show several impressive reflexes that disappear as the child matures. For example, a newborn baby will clasp its fists so tightly around a rope that it can hang on even while being pulled into the air by the rope.

A light tap on the cheek or chin will cause a young infant to rotate its head and open its mouth. This reflex movement helps the baby find a nipple in order to nurse. Such reflexes occur initially whether the baby is awake or asleep but gradually disappear as the child matures.

The fact that anencephalic infants (those born without a cerebrum) show these reflexes indicate that the reflexes arise in lower parts of the brain. Although such reflexes disappear as normal individuals grow up, they sometimes reappear in cerebrum-damaged adults. Given the extreme complexity of the human brain and of human behaviour, it isn't surprising that much of the potential activity is normally suppressed.

And since the learning ability of vertebrates seems to increase with an increase in relative size of the cerebrum, it is not surprising that the cerebrum dominates other regions by suppressing their activity.

Motor Coordination

The *cerebellum*, the second largest part of the brain, superficially resembles the cerebrum in that the surface is folded. But functionally the two regions are totally different. The cerebellum integrates detailed sensory data concerning contraction of muscles and body position with motor commands from the cerebrum.

Actions by the cerebellum permit an individual to carry out smooth, coordinated movements. With cerebellar damage, movements disintegrate into exaggerated components. For example, a normal walk is reduced to a stumbling gait.

The Sensory Filter

Although we may think of the brainstem as a throughway for traffic to higher centers, it is also the site of a web of neurons known as the *reticular formation*. Here sensory impulses are monitored. Obviously, the cerebrum cannot consider all stimuli. It must concentrate on only a few at a time and ignore the others. The reticular formation that receives fibers from every sensory organ screens the sensory data and determines those to be transmitted to the cerebrum.

Control Centers for Fundamental Activities

The *hypothalamus*, which lies deep in the forebrain, controls certain basic behaviours. This control can be demonstrated by electrical stimulation of specific hypothalamic regions. Mild shocks from electrodes in one place will evoke behaviour recognised as evidence of hunger. Animals stimulated in other regions will show thirst, rage, or sexual arousal.

In addition to drives that result in overt activity, the hypothalamus is the center for regulation of internal body functions through autonomic responses. For example, the temperature center lies in the hypothalamus. The fundamental role of the hypothalamus is underscored by the fact that it links the nervous system with the endocrine docrine glands.

The hypothalamus is often considered part of the *limbic system*, a ring-shaped group of centers that lie in the base of the forebrain. Damage to these centers is reflected in alterations of the emotions and changes in the sense of well-being.

The *medulla*, which lies at the junction of the brainstem and the spinal cord, controls such essential life functions as breathing and heart action. For this reason, serious injuries to the medulla end in death. Reflex centers for vomiting, coughing, hiccoughing, and swallowing are also located in the medulla.

Learning and Memory

The physical basis of memory and the changes that occur when animals "*learn*" still elude scientists. Human experience shows that there are at least two kinds of memory. One is quite short-term. It permits us to remember a fact only briefly-for instance, a phone number long enough to ring it.

Other experiences may be remembered over a hundred years of life. The distinction between longterm and short-term memory is readily evident in some aged individuals who can remember details of their childhood but can't recall the events of yesterday.

It has been suggested that short-term learning may result from the initiation of nerve impulses that then reverberate through the "learned" neural circuits. Experimentation with cerebrocortical neurons shows that they exhibit continued electrical activity long after stimulation has ceased.

Whether or not continuous activity is involved in short-term memory, it seems unlikely that such a mechanism could account for the long-term memory that can survive anesthesia, electric shock treatments, and other physical assaults that temporarily interrupt higher brain functions.

To explain long-term memory, many scientists have turned to molecular theories. One popular explanation involves the production of chemicals in which information is coded in much the same manner as genetic information is known to be stored in the DNA of chromosomes. Some scientists have been able to demonstrate the transfer of learning from one animal to another by feeding or injecting chemical extracts of the nervous system of trained organisms.

Other experiments have shown that when goldfish learn a specific task, new proteins of particular kinds accumulate in their brains. Some explanations of long-term memory involve alterations in the properties of synapses or even the establishment of new synapses. Despite much study, no widely accepted explanation has emerged.

Memory seems to be a function of the cerebral cortex in general. Surgical removal of various regions of the cortex from experimental animals gradually decreases learning, but no specific areas have proved crucial. However, stimulation with electrodes implanted in the human cerebral cortex sometimes evokes vivid memories.

THE AUTONOMIC NERVOUS SYSTEM

We have left the autonomic "nervous system" for last, partly because it isn't a simple anatomical part but, instead, involves many different regions. Nevertheless, the autonomic system deserves special attention, because it controls actions independent of our consciousness and because its actions are crucial for homeostasis.

Through motor nerves to the intestines, heart, blood vessels, and other internal organs, the autonomic nervous system regulates activities we could not consciously monitor every minute of the day and night. As noted earlier, autonomic centers lie in the hypothalamus.

A unique characteristic of the autonomic nervous system is its pattern of dual innervation. Almost all organs that receive autonomic fibers have two kinds of fibers. One stimulates activity, and the other inhibits the organ.

Thus the autonomic nervous system provides mechanisms to either speed up or slow down nearly every internal function. Nevertheless, it is incorrect to characterise either of the two parts of the autonomic system (sympathetic or parasympathetic) as being stimulatory or inhibitory. Instead, each division adjusts the body for a particular sort of situation.

The Sympathetic Division

In general, sympathetic stimulation primes the body for crises. Any sudden scare brings on a sympathetic "flight or fight" response. The heart pounds, blood pressure rises, and the bronchioles of the lungs expand as we gasp deeply for air.

At the same time the blood sugar rises, blood vessels in skeletal muscles dilate, and digestive functions are depressed. The body is poised for action. Most terminal axons of the sympathetic system secrete *norepinephrine*. The *adrenal medulla*, usually included as one of the endocrine glands, also produces norepinephrine along with a similar compound, *epinephrine*, also known as adrenalin.

Secretion of closely related chemicals by sympathetic neurons and by the adrenal medulla is a reflection of their common embryonic origin. Furthermore, the adrenal medulla secretes in response to sympathetic stimulation. These facts support the argument that neural and endocrine mechanisms are fundamentally similar.

The Parasympathetic Division

As noted, sympathetic stimulation predominates under stressful circumstances. Parasympathetic stimulation produces the opposite effect. The heartbeat is retarded, breathing is slowed, and digestive juices flow readily. If the sympathetic system is to be remembered for the "fight or flight" response, then we should think of the parasympathetic system in terms of a "*contented cow*" adjustment.

Many basic differences underlie the contrast between the sympathetic and parasympathetic portions of the autonomic nervous system. As we have already mentioned, the sympathetic neurons exert their action through secretion of norepinephrine. In contrast, parasympathetic neurons secrete acetylcholine.

Another difference is that sympathetic fibers arise from spinal nerves along the middle of the cord, but parasympathetic nerves come from the brain or from the lower end of the spinal cord. As an example of autonomic activity, we will examine control of heart rate.

Autonomic Control of Heart Rate

As we pointed out earlier, heart muscle contracts even if all nerves to it are severed. However, the rate of contraction is normally modified by the autonomic nervous system and provides a good example of autonomic involvement in homeostasis. This regulation of heart rate occurs in relation to blood pressure. The amount of blood the heart pumps into the arteries is one factor that determines arterial blood pressure. The faster the heart pumps, the higher the blood pressure. The slower the heart pumps, the lower the blood pressure.

Control of heart rate involves an autonomic reflex. Sympathetic and parasympathetic nerves from centers in the medulla constitute the motor portion of this reflex. The sensory part of the reflex originates in sense organs that measure pressure in the walls of large arteries. Pressure in these arteries stimulates sensory neurons that increase activity of the *cardiac inhibitory center.*

Parasympathetic nerves from this center in the medulla therefore secrete more acetylcholine and thereby slow heart contraction. The same sensory nerves that stimulate the cardiac inhibitory center also inhibit the cardiac accelerator center. Since sympathetic neurons from the *cardiac accelerator center* release epinephrine (adrenalin) that speeds the heart, slowing the accelerator center slows the heart.

In other words, increased pressure in the arteries increases parasympathetic stimulation of the heart and decreases sympathetic stimulation at the same time. Just the opposite occurs as arterial blood pressure falls.

Decreases in arterial blood pressure reduces sensory input to the cardiac centers in the medulla. When the cardiac inhibitor center receives less stimulation, parasympathetic impulses to the heart are reduced. There is now less acetylcholine to slow heart contractions. Less inhibition of the cardiac accelerator center results in increased sympathetic stimulation of the heart.

With more epinephrine, the rate of heart contractions increases. Ordinarily the heart rate results from a balance between parasympathetic stimulation, which slows the heart, and sympathetic stimulation, which speeds it up. Increases in blood pressure reduce sympathetic stimulation and increase parasympathetic stimulation.

Decreases in pressure, increase sympathetic stimulation and decrease parasympathetic stimulation. This pattern of dual controls with opposite actions is characteristic of the autonomic nervous system.

The homeostatic functions of the autonomic nervous system are only one aspect of the general role of the nervous system. That role is to permit the organism to respond to its environment. The response may involve a temporary adjustment of internal organs through the autonomic system.

Or the response may require movement ranging from reflex withdrawal of a hand from a painful stimulus to thoughtfully planned strategies to be carried out over months or years. Whatever the details, the nervous system allows the individual to respond to stimuli.

Repair in the Nervous System

Once nerve cells develop their specialised characteristics, they lose the ability to divide. Nor are there any reserve cells that can replace the old nerve cells. Unlike most other tissues, the nerve cells must last a lifetime. And last they do, unless subjected to unusual damage.

The common tale that we lose a certain percentage of our brain cells every year has not withstood careful examination. The brain shrinks with age, but measurement of the amount of DNA which should reflect numbers of nuclei and hence of cells, seems to remain constant. When there is injury to the nervous system, repair is sometimes possible.

Because peripheral nerves contain nerve fibers but not cell bodies, a severed nerve may repair itself. When a nerve is cut, the neuronal fibers within it degenerate, often as far back as the cell bodies. Then, after a period of recuperation, the damaged cells send out new fibers in the direction of the original connection.

In the meanwhile, any myelin sheath that was there originally has degenerated, but some sheath cells survive and multiply to form a cord of cells. Each new fiber tip probes along the pathway marked by the sheath cells. Growing at 1-2 mm per day, the new fibers often reestablish their original connections.

Surgical techniques that bring the cut ends of a nerve together increase the likelihood that the new fibers will find their way and restore feeling or muscle control. Since new fibers tend to follow the original pathway, the function of the sheath seems important. Nevertheless, how the fibers find their way is not fully understood.

Regeneration of peripheral nerves is seldom complete. Sometimes scar tissue gets in the way of emerging fibers, and they tangle up. Sensory fibers that fail to reach their sense organ may twist into extremely sensitive and painful lumps.

Recovery from peripheral nerve damage can involve more than regeneration of damaged fibers. In at least some cases, surviving neurons sprout new branches that make connections that tend to replace those lost when other fibers are severed. For example, muscle cells with interrupted motor nerves may be reinnervated by branches of neurons that originally served only adjacent muscle cells.

Since repair in peripheral nerves occurs regularly, although imperfectly, it might be expected that repair would also occur normally in the central nervous system. Unfortunately for those who suffer "broken" necks or "broken" backs, this is not so. Spinal cord fibers that are torn

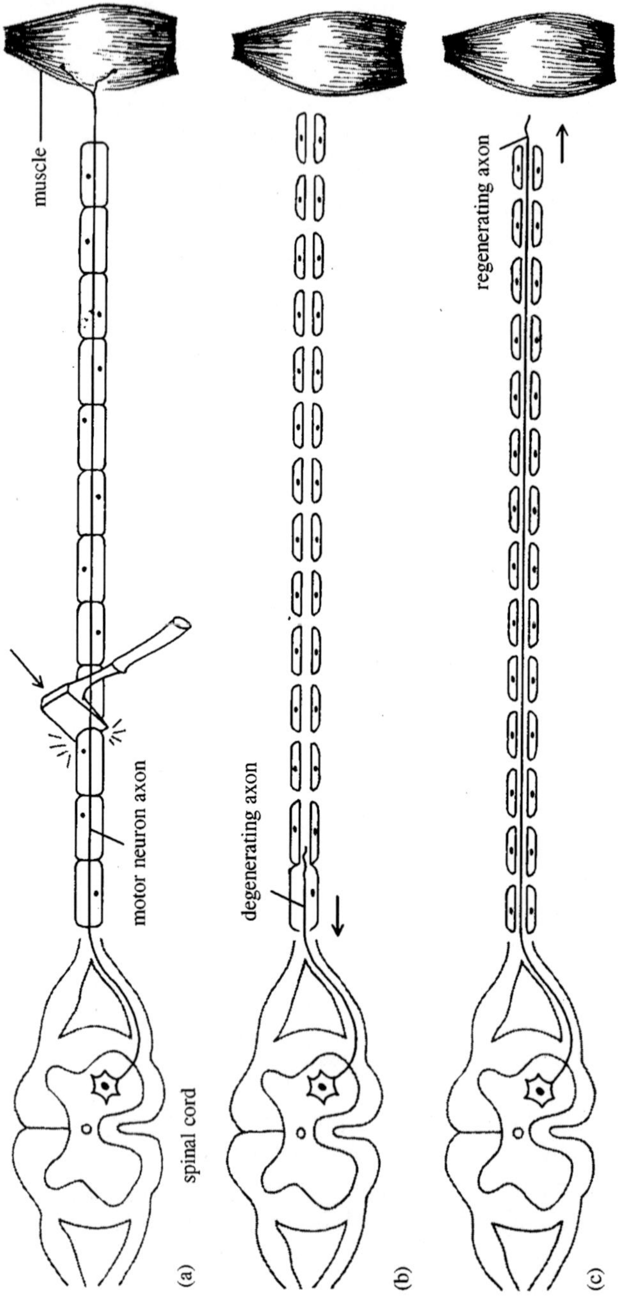

Figure 9.12 : Nerve Regeneration.

when there is damage to neck or trunk vertebrae never heal. It is true that individuals sometimes suffer a temporary paralysis due to spinal injury.

In these cases the fibers aren't severed, but instead, the cells are injured by pressure or temporary lessening of blood flow. With time the injured cells may recover and function normally. But when fibers are broken, the damage is permanent.

Studies with laboratory animals show that injured fibers in the central nervous system grow out, but they don't establish connections. It has frequently been suggested that scar tissue blocks the fibers from reaching the proper point.

It has also been demonstrated that uninjured fibers branch and replace some connections of lost fibers in the brain. Whether or not new connections are a factor in recovery of humans from brain damage has yet to be determined. But many stroke victims do learn to walk and talk after losing these abilities.

Clearly not all brain injuries are hopeless. One encouraging fact is that regeneration has been demonstrated in limited areas of the brains of fish and of frog tadpoles. It has also been shown in one tiny area of a mammalian brain.

Organisation for Response

Although species without distinct nerve cells exhibit specific response patterns, most animals have specialised cells we recognise as neurons. The simplest organisation of neurons is found in coelenterates. As shown in Figure elsewhere in this chpater, jellyfish and other coelenterates have a saclike body.

The single opening of the sac is the central organisational feature of the body. This body pattern is an example of *radial symmetry*. (The circular body can be cut along radii into several equal pie-shaped wedges.) With radial symmetry any point on the periphery can take the lead when the organism moves.

There is no single best location for tissues that coordinate response to newly encountered stimuli. In other words, there is no head and no brain. Since there is no standard orientation for responses, one-way nerve pathways would be disadvantageous. Thus synapses in coelenterates can transmit impulses in either direction. The coelenterate nervous system can best be described as a network of cells. Since synapses transmit in either direction, stimulation at any location results in a generalised response that spreads gradually in all directions.

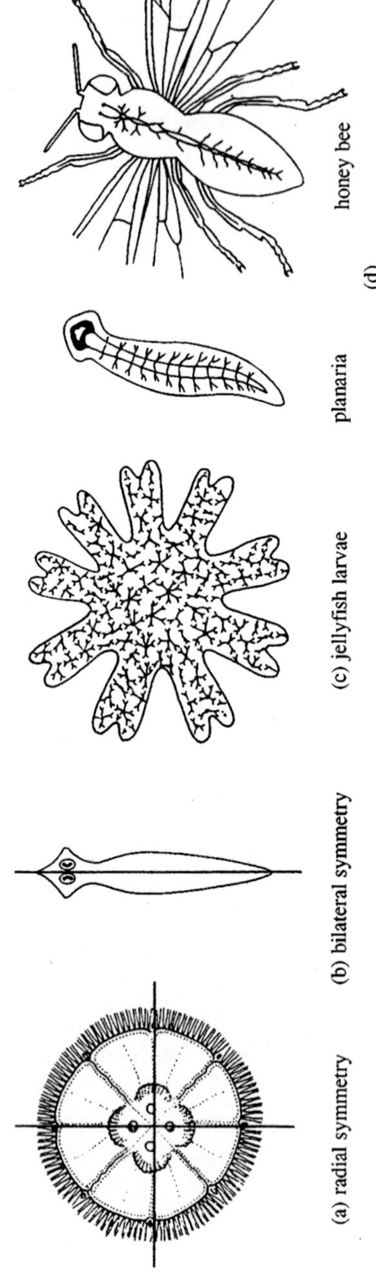

Figure 9.13 : How body plan determines organisation of the nervous system.

In contrast to the radial symmetry of coelenterates, most animals are *bilaterally symmetrical*. Each has a head and can be divided into similar parts only by a single plane that separates the body into mirror-image right and left halves. Bilaterally symmetrical animals move headfirst.

The concentration of sense organs and nervous system in the head is an efficient organisation that has been favoured by natural selection. Although the nervous systems of worms, insects, and other bilaterally symmetrical animals vary, all are fundamentally similar. Each has a brain, each has a nerve cord that extends posteriorly from the head, and each has one-way synapses.

Although most multicellular animals have neurons, such specialised cells are unnecessary for response to stimuli. Consider the example of bacteria that swim toward an oxygen source despite the absence of any coordinating structure. In fact, *irritability*, the property of responding to stimuli, is characteristic of all organisms, including green plants and fungi.

HORMONES AND THE BRAIN

As we have seen, nerve action relies on the secretion of chemical messengers by neurons. However, neurotransmitters carry information only a short distance, specifically across the synaptic gap between axon and dendrite. Other chemical messengers of the body usually work at a distance from their point of origin.

These are the *hormones* secreted by *endocrine tissues*. It is customary to speak of an *endocrine system*, but this system is not comparable to the digestive or nervous system in that it is not structurally united. Instead, the components of the endocrine system are scattered about the body. They constitute a system only in that they share some modes of operation and are responsible for important aspects of homeostatic regulation.

Many endocrine tissues occur as large masses of glandular tissue named as distinct organs. Other endocrine cells are hidden in organs better known for other functions. Examples include intestinal cells that produce the digestive hormones secretin and enterogastrone.

But no matter what the exact organisation of endocrine tissues is, their secretions enter the blood. Because the blood distributes hormones throughout the body, there is no need for endocrine glands to have ducts. Unlike glands that secrete lubricating fluids or digestive enzymes, endocrine glands are ductless.

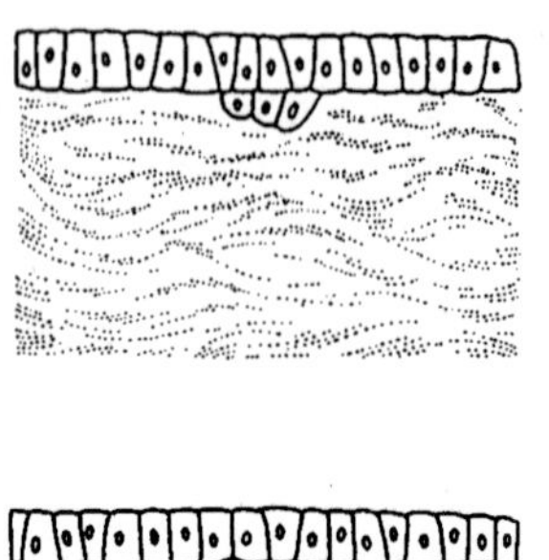

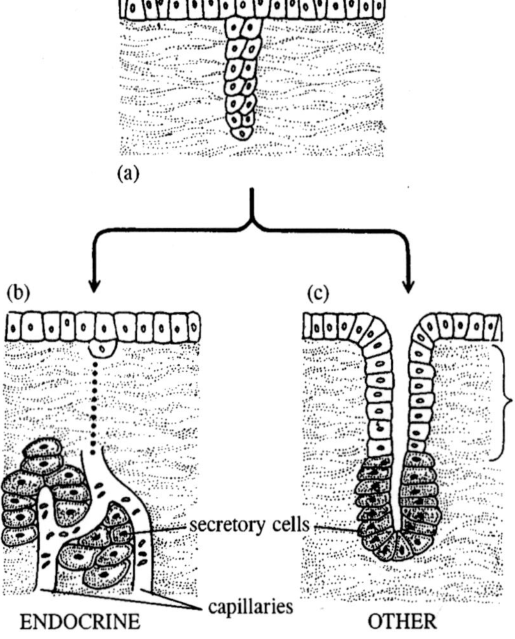

Figure 9.14 : How endocrine glands develop without ducts all.

Although all the organs of the body come into contact with most hormones, in many cases only one or a few kinds of *target cells* actually respond to a particular hormone.

Hormones generally control characteristic life patterns and make relatively slow, gradual adjustments. Thus hormones regulate growth, sexual development and activity, the water content of the body, the metabolic rate, and some aspects of digestion. By way of contrast, nerves are responsible for mainly rapid changes. Our nervous system permits us to respond to our environment and manipulate it. Nerves largely regulate muscles, both the skeletal muscles that move our bones and internal muscles, such as those of the heart and blood vessels. Any attempt to divide neural and hormonal activities blurs, of course, as we have already seen in our discussion of the effect of adrenal hormones on the heart muscle. But the complex relationship between the nervous system and the endocrine system doesn't end here. Ultimately, the nervous system controls most endocrine glands.

THE HYPOTHALAMIC-PITUITARY AXIS

The *pituitary*, a pea-sized gland, lies at the base of the brain just below the hypothalamus. Here it is protected in a bony pocket of the skull. The pituitary consists of distinct anterior and posterior lobes.The posterior lobe of the pituitary is attached by a stalk to the hypothalamus and is really part of the brain.

In fact, hormones released by the *posterior pituitary*, such as antidiuretic hormone, are synthesized in the cell bodies of neurons within the hypothalamus. These hormones pass along axons of the hypothalamic cells into the posterior pituitary, where they are stored for later release.

The posterior pituitary is merely a projection of the brain itself, but the *anterior pituitary* is distinctly different. The cells of the anterior pituitary lack neuronal characteristics, and this gland originates from the roof of the mouth and is connected to the brain only by blood vessels. It is the anterior pituitary that is sometimes called the "*master gland*" of the body.

Through hormone secretion the anterior pituitary controls the activities of the thyroid, adrenals, and sex glands. Furthermore, an anterior pituitary hormone controls growth. Nevertheless, the hypothalamus determines to a large extent the activity of the anterior pituitary.

Although the hormones of the anterior pituitary are secreted within the gland itself, these hormones are released only when the anterior pituitary is stimulated by *releasing factors* produced by the hypothalamus. A special network of blood vessels carries blood from the hypothalamus directly to the anterior pituitary. Through these vessels the releasing factors reach the anterior pituitary.

Perhaps dependence of the endocrine system on the nervous system should be expected. After all, it is the nervous system that receives stimuli from outside the body and hence is in a position to determine the proper level of activities of other internal organs.

Feedback Control

Do you recall the discussion of feedback control of enzymes in othr

Table 9.2 : Endocrine Glands and Hormone Actions

Gland	Hormone	Effects
I. HORMONES ASSEMBLED MAINLY OF AMINO ACIDS		
Adrenal medulla	**Epinephrine** (also known as adrenalin)	Generally stimulates the same functions that are promoted by nerve impulses from the sympathetic portion of the autonomic nervous system.
Anterior pituitary	**Adrenal corticotropic hormone** (ACTH)	Promotes secretion of glucocorticoids by the adre-nal cortex.
	Follicle-stimulating hormone (FSH)	In females, stimulates growth of ovarian follicles and estrogen secretion; in males, development of seminiferous tubules and sperm formation.
	Growth hormone (GH)	Promotes skeletal and gene-ral body growth.
	Luteinizing hormone (LH, also known as interstitial-cell-stimulating hormone or ICSH in males)	In females, promotes ovulation and develoment and maintenance of the corpus luteum; in males, testosterone secretion and sperm release.
	Prolactin	Promotes milk secretion by mammary glands after childbirth.
	Thyroid-stimulating tract cells	Stimulates closure of pyloric sphincter between stomach and small intestine.
	Choleocystokinin	Stimulates the gall bladder to release its contents into the small intestine.
	Gastrin	Stimulates release of digestive enzymes from small intestine.
	Secretin	Stimulates pancreas to secrete sodium bicarbonate into the small intestine.
Hypo-thalamus	**Adrenal corticotropic releasing factor (CRF)**	Stimulates release of ACTH.
	Follicle-stimulating hormone releasing factor (FSHRF)	Stimulates release of LH.

Gland	Hormone	Effects
	Growth hormone re-leasing factor (GHRF)	Stimulates release of GH.
	Luteinizing hormone re-leasing factor (LHRF)	Stimulates release of LH.
	Prolactin releasing fac-for (PRF)	Stimulates release of prolactin.
	Thyroid-stimulating hormone releasing fac-tor (TSHRF)	Stimulates release of TSH.
Pancreas	**Glucagon**	Promotes conversion of glyco-gen to glucose.
	Insulin	Promotes conversion of glucose to glycogen; facilitates passage of glucose across cell memb-ranes.
Para-thyroid	**Parathyroid hormone**	Increases blood calcium by promoting intestinal absorption of calcium, calcium reabsor-ption from bone, and retention of calcium in the kidneys.
Placenta	**Chorionic gonadotropin**	Maintains health of the corpus luteum, even in absence of LH.
Posterior pituitary (hormones actually	**Antidiuretic hormone (ADH)**	Promotes water re absorption in the kidney and keeps urine volume small.
from hypo-thalamus)	Oxytocin (also known as pitressin, or "pit")	Stimulates childbirth and release of milk from mammary glands afterwards.
Thyroid	**Calcitonin**	Decreases blood calcium by opposing activities promoted by parathyroid hormone.
	Thyroxin and related hormones	Increases cellular respiration and protein synthesis.
II. STEROID HORMONES		
Adrenal cortex	**Aldosterone**	Regulates sodium and potassium levels and thereby blood volume

Gland	Hormone	Effects
		and blood pressure.
	Estrogen	See below.
	Glucocorticoids (such as cortisol, which the body converts to the better-known hormone cortisone)	Promotes synthesis of glucose from amino acids and fats; inhibits inflammation and allergic reactions.
	Testosterone	See below.
Ovary	**Estrogen**	In females, stimulates growth of uterine muscle and of mammary glands during pregnancy; development of uterine lining during monthly cycle; also secondary sexual characteristics, such as fat deposits in skin, especially on hips and breasts.
	Progesterone	In females, stimulates development of uterus and breast during pregnancy; development of uterine lining during monthly cycle.
	Testosterone	In females, function is not clear; can promote male secondary sex characteristics, such as increased facial hair when excessive or not balanced by estrogen.
Placenta	**Estrogen**	See above.
	Progesterone	See above.
Testis	**Estrogen**	In males, function is not clear; see above.
	Testosterone	In males, stimulates sperm production and male secondary characteristics, including facial hair.

Chapter of this book. It turns out that the production of many hormones is regulated by a similar but somewhat more complex arrangement in which the hypothalamus plays a key role.

Here is the usual pattern.The hypothalamus normally secretes a specific releasing factor that stimulates the anterior pituitary to produce a particular hormone. The target organ for this pituitary hormone is another endocrine gland that responds by secreting its characteristic hormone, which produces a useful physiological effect.

An increase in the blood concentration of this final hormone beyond a critical level inhibits secretion of the releasing factor by the hypothalamus. This, in turn, stops secretion of that particular pituitary hormone and ultimately shuts down the second endocrine gland. This explanation is illustrated by the relationship between the hypothalamus, pituitary, and thyroid.

Thyroid-stimulating hormone releasing factor (TSHRF) from the hypothalamus causes the anterior pituitary to secrete *thyroid-stimulating hormone* (TSH), which causes the thyroid to produce *thyroxin*. The presence of thyroxin in the blood of the hypothalamus inhibits production of TSHRF and thus limits secretion of thyroxin.

Because thyroxin regulates cellular respiration and hence the heat available to maintain our body temperature, this system must be adjusted to meet long-term fluctuations in environmental temperatures. We receive the first cool breezes of fall as if they were wintery blasts, partly because our metabolism is still set for summer conditions.

But after a few weeks the hypothalamus responds to decreased environmental temperatures by secreting more TSHRF. As a result, thyroxin production increases, cellular respiration is accelerated, and we are comfortable at temperatures several degrees cooler than we could accept previously. Feedback control involving the hypothalamus, anterior pituitary, and reproductive hormones will be discussed in othr Chapter of this book.

HOW HORMONES WORK

As diverse as hormones are, most seem to exert their action on particular target cells by one or the other of two methods. Hormones that are steroids" (mainly secretions of the adrenal cortex, ovary, and testis) penetrate the cell membrane and bind to nuclear components. It seems likely that the activity of these hormones involves a somewhat direct regulation of the action of genes.

The nonsteroid hormones are proteins or related smaller compounds

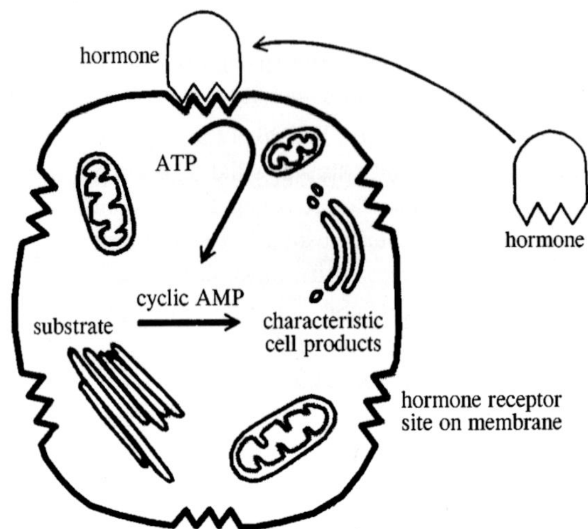

Figure 9.15 : Cyclic AMP as a Second Messenger.

made up of amino acids or modified amino acids. These hormone messengers bind to specific receptors on the cell membrane. The binding activates an enzyme located in the membrane and causes the enzyme to manufacture an internal or second messenger.

One such messenger is **cAMP** (cyclic adenosine monophosphate) which is produced from ATP. Increased cAMP stimulates cell activity. Exactly which activity increases, however, depends on the nature of the cell. For example, cAMP causes pancreatic cells to secrete glucagon, but it stimulates thyroid cells to produce thyroxin and liver cells to convert glycogen into glucose.

Thus cAMP is a second messenger, which serves as a relay between the hormone that stops at the cell membrane and metabolic activity within the cell.

A LOOK AT THE WHOLE

Important as they are, neurons and endocrine cells can't regulate our internal environment by themselves. You will recall that reflex control of heart rate required sense organs that measure pressure in the arteries. Similarly, the hypothalamus-pituitary-thyroid system for regulating metabolism responds to input from temperature sensors.

It seems obvious that mechanisms for maintaining a constant internal environment require information about both internal and external conditions. In addition, many adjustments of our external environment rely on skeletal muscles. Similarly, adjustments of our internal environment may involve muscle of the intestine or other internal organs. In reality, both sense organs and muscles are components of our homeostatic apparatus.

10

REPRODUCTION

Two topics have universal appeal. One is sex and the other is the development of babies. Probably this appeal has a deep biological basis. After all, these processes are the immediate keys to the continued existence of our species. People without much interest in either topic aren't very likely to contribute to the next generation.

This chapter is about sexual reproduction. You are surely aware that although everyone is interested in sex, it is still a controversial subject. During your earlier schooling you may have been "*protected*" from some of the information we present here.

This isn't surprising, since so many aspects of sex have social significance as well as emotional impact. For example, there is the matter of differences between men and women and how they affect traditional sex roles. There are also questions concerning contraception, *abortion*, *homosexuality*, and *sexual sensations*. The very mention of these topics threatens some people.

But we believe everyone should have access to accurate information. Unfortunately, research into sexuality is relatively new, and there is still much to learn. Most people experience difficulty in studying this topic objectively. Try to treat it as you have other aspects of human biology. Death by accident, disease or aging awaits al organisms.

So, if a population is to continue, those that die must be replaced. Reproductive mechanisms are as diverse as species, but even though we uswually associate reproduction and sex, some species can reproduce asexually. In asexual reproduciton a single parent produces offspring with characteristics identical to itself. This method has important advantages. For one, it isn't dependent on the presence of other individuals.

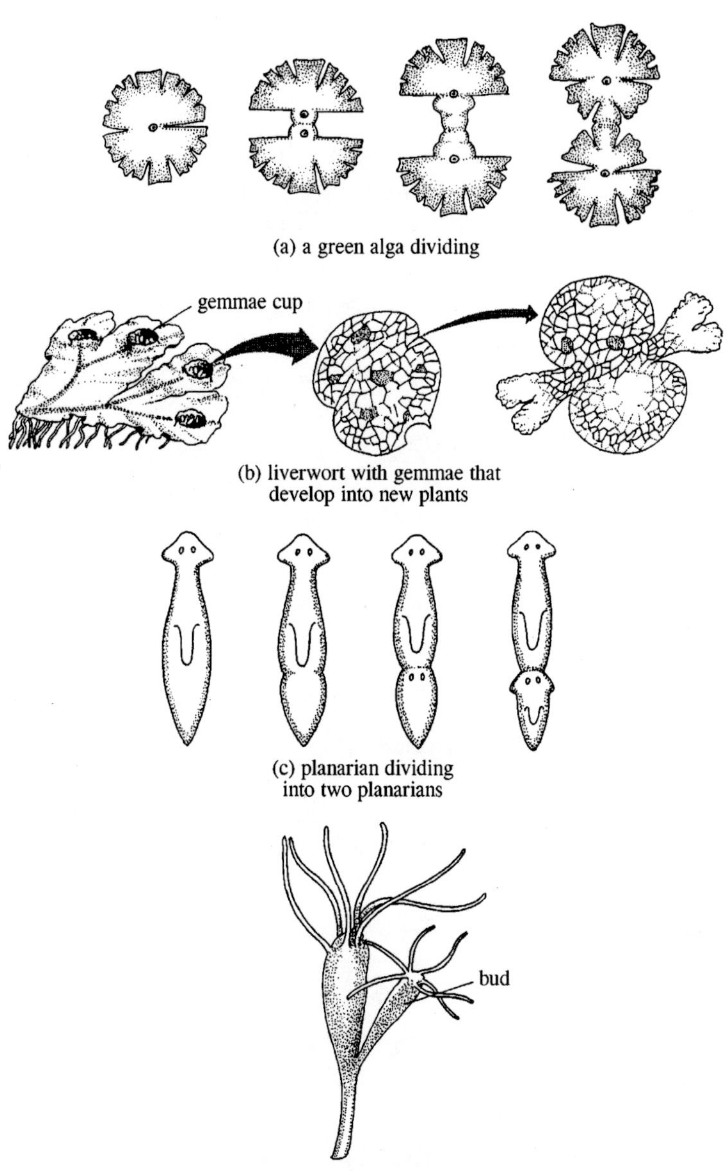

Figure 10.1 : Asexual Reproduction.

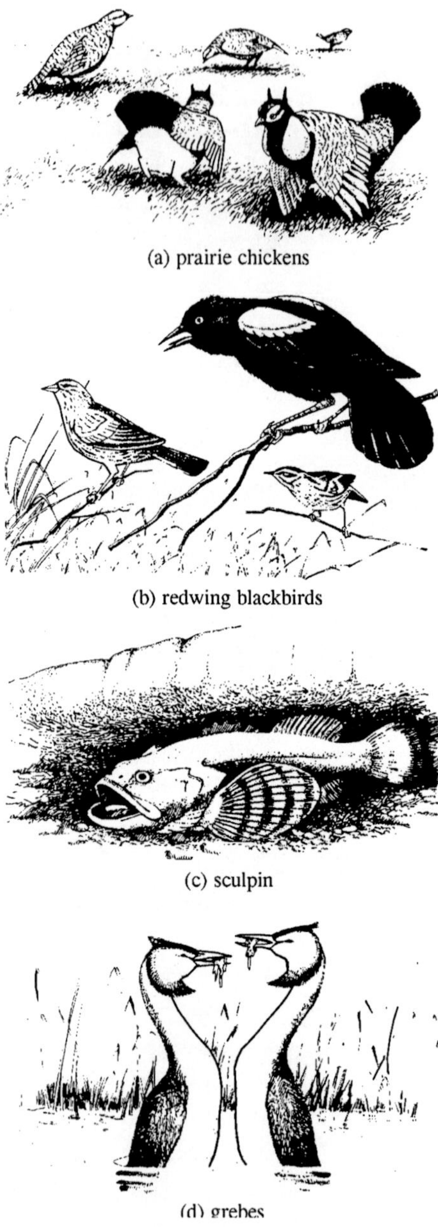

(a) prairie chickens

(b) redwing blackbirds

(c) sculpin

(d) grebes

Figure 10.2 : Courtship is serious business.

One organism can start a whole new population. Furthermore, asexual reproduction may be simpler and more efficient. By comparision, sexual reproduction may seem needlessly complicated.

SEX: WHAT AND WHY

Sexual reproduction involves fusion of cells from two individuals. For most species these individuals and their sex cells differ. *Males* produce small, actively motile cells called *sperm*. In contrast, the *female* egg, or *ovum*, is a large cell rich in food reserves and cytoplasmic organelles. It cannot move actively; it can only drift or be carried by action of surrounding cells.

To form a new individual, the sperm and egg must meet. Elaborate structures and complex behaviour can be necessary to bring about this union. The midnight brawls of cats, the spring chorus of frogs, the nesting-season music of song birds, and myriad courtship displays all contribute to bringing sperm and eggs together.

For humans the interest, emotion, and drive that surround sex serve the same purpose, to ensure that sperm reach eggs. The love of children and the desire to have them are a powerful force in many human lives. Nevertheless, what people often seek in sex is personal gratification, companionship, love, or maybe just escape. In our culture the psychological and social consequences of sex blur its biological significance. But in the bargain we beget and conceive children.

Compared with asexual reproduction, sexual reproduction may seem cumbersome. Nevertheless, the vast majority of organisms reproduce by sexual means-and for good reason. Sexual reproduction does not merely preserve the old patterns. Union of hereditary material in the egg and sperm produces young that are different from either parent.

Thus every new generation of a sexually reproducing species contains new combinations of characteristics. This increases the chance that the species can survive any environmental changes. It is for this reason that species that usually reproduce asexually almost always have sexual reproduction as well. Sometimes asexual and sexual reproduction are both part of one life cycle. Other species, including all mammals,' are strictly sexual creatures.

MAN: SPECIALISATION FOR TRANSFER OF GENETIC MATERIAL

The reproductive system of human males consists of an extensive complex of glands and tubes, together with the *external genitals*, the penis and scrotum. The tube system begins in the testes, where it is the

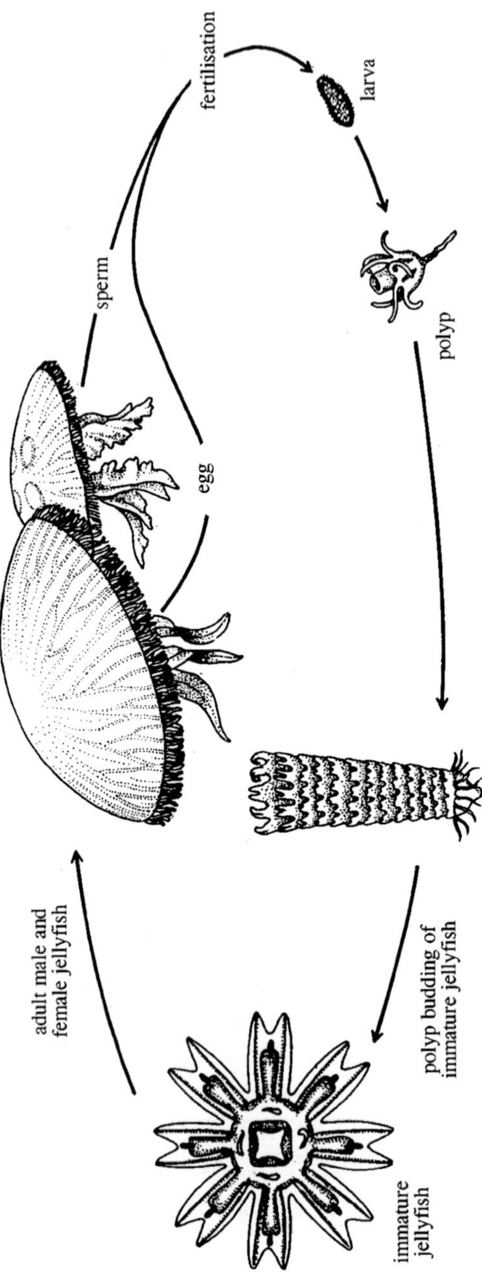

Figure 10.3 : Sexual and Asexual Reproduction Alternate in Jellyfish.

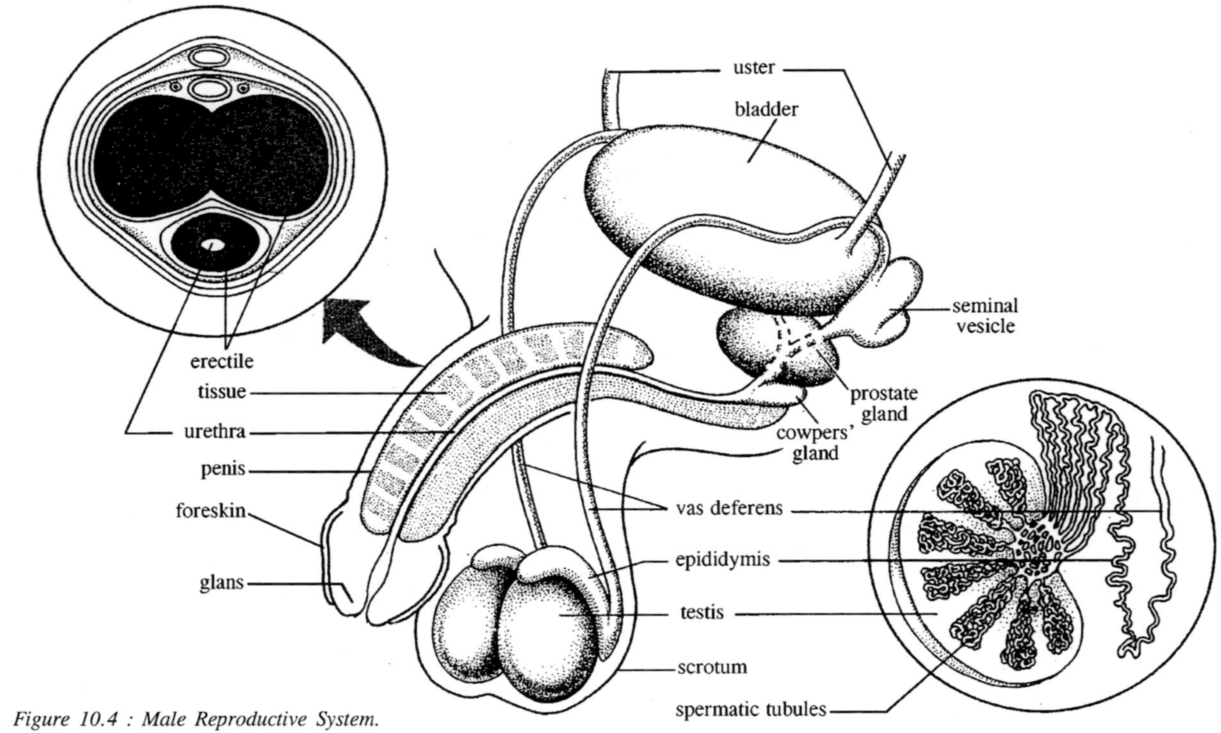

Figure 10.4 : Male Reproductive System.

site of sperm production, and extends to the penis. Along the way, five glands secrete fluids that contribute to the semen.

The Testes

The testes are the male *gonads*, that is, the source of the male sex cells. In men these sperm-producing organs lie within the *scrotum*, a pouch of skin that hangs behind the penis. The scrotum is normally quite loose, but when a man is cold or frightened, muscle in the skin contracts and tightens the scrotum, pulling it closer to the body.

To reach the scrotum, the testes migrate from their point of origin near the kidneys, usually during the last two months before birth. As the testes descend into the scrotum, they pass through the *inguinal canals*, openings in the abdominal wall. Blood vessels and nerves serving each testis and its sperm duct (vas deferens) follow the descending testis and lie in the canals thereafter.

These canals between muscles of the abdominal wall are weak spots that can be opened by pressure. Lifting or straining may rupture the wall and force a loop of intestine into a canal, producing an *inguinal hernia*.

The normal location of the testes in the scrotum, rather than deep in the body cavity, seems related to heat sensitivity of the sperm-producing tissue. If the testes remain in the body cavity, the heat there will destroy the germinal tissue. Although testes often fail to descend properly, sterility can be prevented through a simple operation on the newborn baby. The testes are drawn from the abdominal cavity to the scrotum, where they belong.

The testes have two main functions: formation of sperm and production of the male sex hormone *testosterone*. Sperm develop in long, coiled *spermatic tubules*. Among the tubules lie *interstitial cells*, which synthesize testosterone. Production of sperm and testosterone are continuous in the male, in contrast to the more cyclic nature of female reproductive events.

Testosterone is necessary for full development of the spermatic tubules and for *libido* (sex drive). It is also responsible for the secondary sexual characteristics of males, including a low voice, heavy facial hair, a muscular body, and distinctive skeletal build. These and other hormonal aspects of sexual differences will be explored when we compare men and women later in this chapter.

Activity of the testis is regulated by pituitary hormones. *Interstitial-cell-stimulating hormone* (ICSH) from the anterior pituitary is necessary for secretion of testosterone by the interstitial cells. *Follicle-stimulating hormone* (FSH-named for its function in the female) supports normal development of spermatic tubules. Through a negative-feedback mechanism involving the hypothalamus, testosterone reduces secretion of ICSH and FSH.

Sperm

Sperm formation begins with special cell divisions during a process known as meiosis. These divisions and their role in the patterns of inheritance will be discussed in other Chapter of this book. For now we will examine only the maturation that converts rather ordinaryappearing immature sperm cells into specialised carriers of genetic information. In this process the nucleus condenses to form the dense sperm head.

At the tip of the head, the *acrosome*, a sac of enzymes develops. Later these enzymes aid in penetration of the egg. Eventually, the scattered mitochondria of the developing sperm become closely packed into a spiral behind the head. This *mitochondrial spiral* is twisted around the root of the flagellum that makes up the long tail.

Arranged this way, the mitochondria require little space but are strategically located to supply energy to the flagellum that propels the sperm. During sperm maturation, much of the original cytoplasm is discarded. The fully developed sperm consists only of a densely packed genetic "payload" and the structures necessary to carry this material to the egg.

Sperm are shed by the spermatic tubules into the *epididymis*, an extensively coiled tube that connects with the *vas deferens* (vessel that carries away; plural, *vasa deferentia*). The vas deferens extends up into the abdominal cavity, where it joins the urethra. Thus the sperm leave the body via the urethra, as does the urine.'

Sperm accumulate in the epididymis and must remain there for at least three weeks before they are completely mature. Although resorption of sperm occurs if the vas deferens is severed surgically, sperm are ordinarily released at intercourse or by masturbation or during nocturnal emissions (wet dreams). When sperm leave the male tract, they are fully motile. However, a further change, triggered by female secretions, is necessary before a sperm can fertilise an egg.

Semen

Before they leave the body, sperm are suspended in glandular secretions. These liquids come mainly from the *seminal vesicles*, the *prostate*, and the *Cowper's glands*. Together these fluids and the suspended sperm make up the milky *semen*, the fluid that is ejaculated from a man's body when he has an orgasm.

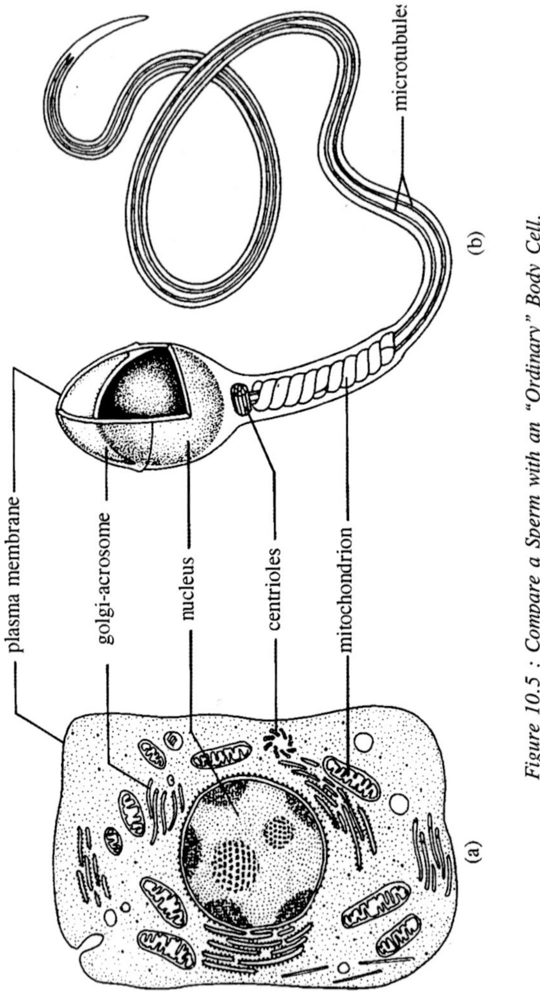

Figure 10.5 : Compare a Sperm with an "Ordinary" Body Cell.

Of the three sets of accessory glands that contribute to the semen, the prostate is the largest. The location of the prostate can prove a treacherous arrangement in older men. It surounds the junction of the vas deferens and the urethra. In many aged males the prostatic tissue recommences growth. Usually-but not always-these growths are noncancerous. Nevertheless, even a simple enlargement of the prostate causes problems. The new growth compresses the urethra, making urination difficult or impossible. Sometimes urine backs up into the kidneys, and the pressure destroys them.

The Penis

The penis provides a conduit for the urethra, which carries urine and semen to the outside of the body. A vertical slit at the tip of the penis marks the opening of the urethra. The skin that covers the outside of the penis shaft is folded back on itself at the tip to form the *foreskin*, which covers the glans. The *glans* is the large, smooth end of the penis that is especially sensitive to stimulation and that enlarges greatly during erection.

Unlike many animals, the human male has no cartilage or bone in the penis. It is normally soft and flaccid. But within the penis lie three masses of erectile tissue that expand with blood during sexual excitement and enlarge and stiffen the penis. One of the bodies of erectile tissue surrounds the urethra and expands at the tip to fill the glans.

WOMAN: CYCLIC CHANGES PERMIT MULTIPLE TASKS

In contrast to the meandering tubes and multiple glands of the male reproductive tract, the female organs appear deceptively simple. They consist of a pair of *ovaries* (female gonads); *Fallopian tubes* (oviducts), which lead to the *uterus* (womb); the *vagina*; and external genitals. Some organs, especially the ovary and uterus, undergo marked cyclic changes. These changes occur as each ovum matures and either degenerates or is fertilised and develops into a baby.

Sperm deposited in the vagina make their way through a tiny opening in the *cervix*, or "neck," at the lower end of the uterus (Fig. 11.8). Fertilisation most often occurs in the Fallopian tubes. The fertilised egg soon begins to divide. Now referred to as an *embryo*, it passes to the uterus, a journey of a few days, and remains there until birth.

Thus the female structures must produce the egg, receive the sperm, permit fertilisation, nurture the new individual as it grows to as much as 10 percent of the mother's body weight, and then expel it alive. Once a month the female reproductive tract begins a cycle of dramatic activities that prepare it for these several different tasks. These activities are regulated by the interactions of a number of hormones.

Ovarian Cycles

A newborn female has hundreds of thousands of partially developed eggs in her ovaries. The ova are in a resting stage; in fact, almost all of them will eventually degenerate. No more than about 400 ova ever ripen to be released from the ovaries. In a sexually mature woman *follicle-stimulating hormone* (FSH) from the pituitary causes several

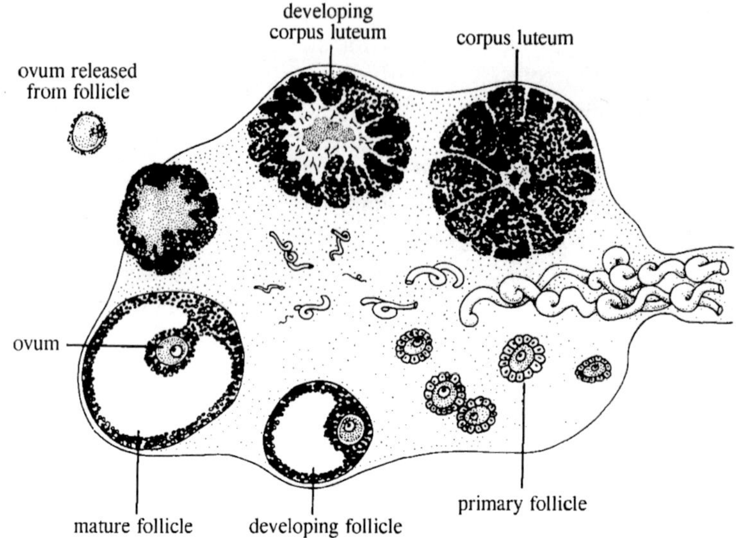

Figure 10.6 : Diagram of the Life of an Ovarian Follicle

ova to resume development each month. As the ova grow, they increase in size without the obvious changes in form seen in sperm development.

Growth of an ovum is accompanied by an ever greater number of *follicle* (nurse) *cells*, surrounding the egg. Although several follicles begin to develop each month, usually only one reaches maturity; the others degenerate. And as a follicle enlarges, it pushes away any smaller follicles that lie between it and the surface of the ovary. Soon the growing follicle forms a blisterlike bulge on the ovary.

Both the ovary and the uterus undergo cyclic changes. Together the hypothalamus and the anterior pituitary control these female reproductive cycles. One or more releasing factors (RF) secreted by the hypothalamus stimulate the secretion of FSH and LH from the anterior pituitary. The FSH promotes development of ovarian follicles containing the ova (eggs).

LH promotes ovulation and development of the follicular remains into a corpus luteum. Estrogen from developing follicles, together with progesterone and estrogen from the corpus luteum, restricts hypothalamic stimulation of the anterior pituitary, as well as promotes development of the uterine lining. The negative influence of ovarian hormones on secretion of FSH and LH brings each cycle to a close. Withdrawal of ovarian hormones causes shedding of the uterine lining (menstruation), as well as permits the hypothalamus to again stimulate the anterior

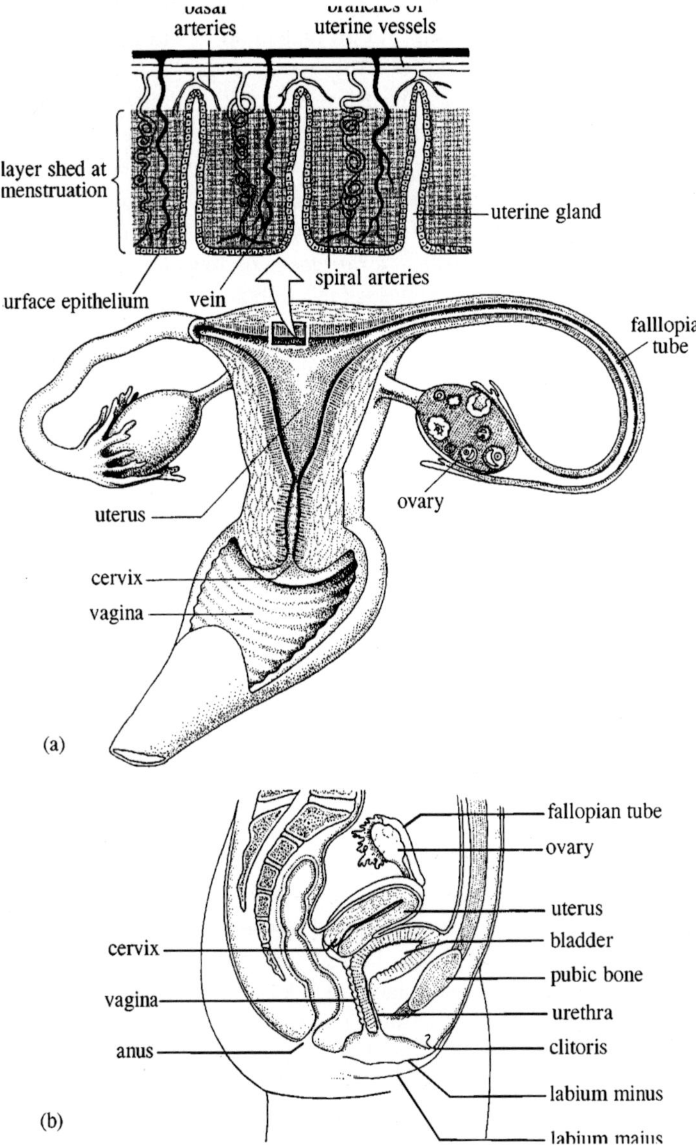

Figure 10.7 : Female reproductive System.

pituitary. On the basis of this information, explain how birth control pills containing estrogen and progesterone prevent conception.

In addition to stimulating the growth of follicles, FSH spurs the nurse cells of the developing follicles to secrete the hormone *estrogen*. But as follicles grow and estrogen levels increase, the larger amounts of estrogen inhibit the activity of the pituitary, so release of FSH declines.

In the absence of sufficient FSH, secretion of estrogen levels off, allowing another surge of FSH. At the same time, the pituitary secretes increasing quantities of *luteinizing hormone*, or LH. Together the high concentrations of LH and FSH cause the follicle to rupture and release the egg. This process is *ovulation*.

Usually only one follicle matures each cycle. Although numerous follicles begin to enlarge at the start of the cycle, most degenerate before the ova are ready to be released.

After Ovulation

The open mouth of the Fallopian tube extends like a bonnet partway around the ovary. Contractions of the oviduct may draw the finger-like edges of the open mouth of the tube over the ovary surface and gather the egg into the oviduct. Once within the oviduct, the egg is moved toward the uterus by cilia lining the walls and by contractions of muscles within the walls.

After the egg has left the ovary, LH causes the cells of the old empty follicle to transform into a *corpus luteum*. The corpus luteum is endocrine tissue; it secretes both estrogen and a second female hormone, *progesterone*. Progesterone inhibits secretion of LH, which is necessary to maintain the corpus luteum. Without LH the corpus luteum dies unless pregnancy occurs. If it does, a placental hormone is secreted that replaces LH.

Death of the corpus luteum, followed by elimination of progesterone and estrogen through the urine, leaves the body with little of either ovarian hormone. As you may have recognised, these hormones exert negative-feedback control over the pituitary secretions that regulate the ovary. In their absence, the pituitary soon recovers its activity and begins to secrete FSH once more.

Actually FSH and LH are produced by the anterior pituitary in response to substances released by the hypothalamus. The inhibitory action of estrogen and progesterone works indirectly through the hypothalamus. Excitement, fear, and other strong emotions frequently alter the normal course of events by their effect on the hypothalamus.

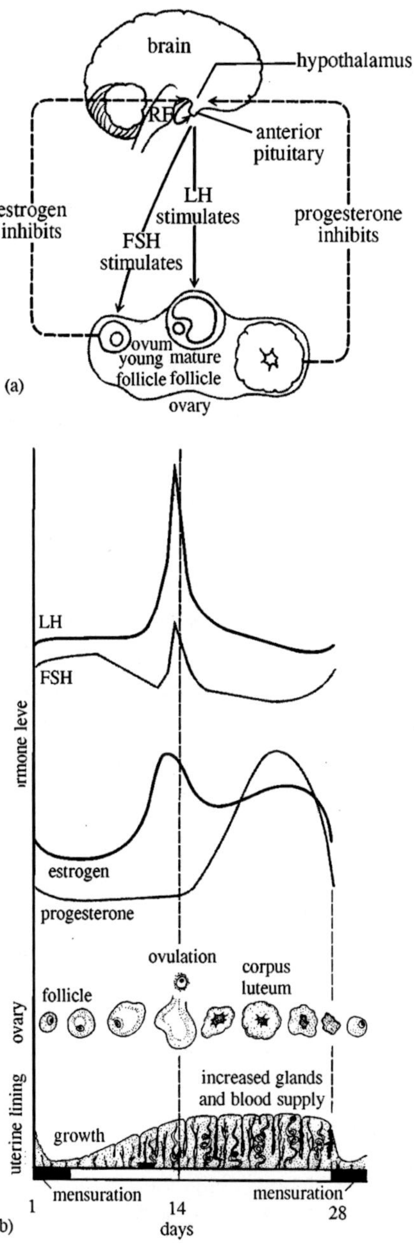

Figure 10.8 : Hormone-Controlled Female Cycles.

Uterine Cycles

Associated with the cyclic changes in hormones are cyclic changes in the uterus. These changes show themselves as the *menstrual*, or monthly, cycle. Estrogen from the growing follicles makes the lining of the uterus thicken. Glands there grow deeper, and blood vessels proliferate. After ovulation, progesterone causes further thickening and enrichment of the uterine tissues.

The glands branch out, and the lining becomes plump with blood. All is ready for a fertilised egg if one appears. In the absence of pregnancy, however, the corpus luteum dies and both estrogen and progesterone levels drop. The uterine lining loses tissue fluids and shrinks. Shrinkage compresses and interrupts blood flow in the spiral arteries that supply the outer layer of the lining.

The walls of the capillaries and veins supplied by these arteries soon die. So do the surrounding tissues. Eventually the outer layer of the uterine lining sloughs off, releasing small amounts of stagnant blood. Normally the arteries heal over before the dead layer falls away. Therefore fresh blood is usually not released. The cells lining the depth of the glands remain when the surface layer is lost.

These gland cells divide to supply additional cells that grow over the raw surface left by menstruation. Before continuing further, study Figure elsewhere in this chapter carefully. Correlate the changes in pituitary and ovarian hormones, the changes in the ovary, and those in the uterus during the entire menstrual cycle.

Most women suffer mild to severe discomfort during menstruation. This discomfort is associated with exaggerated uterine contractions, now believed due to excess prostaglandins. Withdrawal of progesterones permits prostaglandins to stimulate uterine contractions. Women who suffer menstrual cramps have excessive prostaglandins in the menstrual discharge.

The pain comes from hard contractions that deprive the working muscle of adequate oxygen. The nausea, headache, and other menstrual symptoms may stem from increased contraction of blood vessel muscles that rob the stomach and brain of adequate blood supply.

The Embryo Supports Itself

During pregnancy the developing embryo produces a hormone that mimics the effects of LH by keeping the corpus luteum in good health. This hormone is named *chorionic gonadotropin* because it is produced by the embryonic membrane known as the chorion and because it affects the ovary (gonad). As long as estrogen is secreted, FSH production is repressed and no further eggs can develop. Later in pregnancy the placenta secretes massive amounts of both estrogen and progesterone.

Menopause

The cyclic oscillations of pituitary and ovarian hormones occur from puberty (sexual maturity) to menopause. At that point, usually late in the fifth decade; hormonal cycles and menstruation cease. The woman's reproductive life, but not her sexual life, is brought to a close.

Menopause results from exhaustion of the ovary, not of the pituitary. In fact, the level of FSH is sometimes elevated during menopause, because estrogen decreases as the number of developing follicles slowly dwindles. Many of the later cycles produce no ova.

LOVEMAKING

Love making, *coitus*, the sex act, sexual relations, intercourse, and numerous slang terms are synonyms for the process biologists usually refer to as *copulation*, or mating. As humans we are interested not only in the anatomical details of this process but also in the physiological bases of the sexual climax known as *orgasm*.

Sexual experiences have both physiological and psychological components. Until recent years prudishness or, perhaps, awe prevented scientific study of the phenomena.

What Happens

As everyone knows, people are different from one another. Probably no two sexual experiences are exactly alike, even for the same individual. But basically a sexual experience involves a gradual and then an explosive increase in tension followed by relaxation. The tension arises from the swelling of tissue with blood and from muscle contractions.

Blood vessel changes occur in many organs, not only those obviously associated with sex. One can direct these changes consciously only by concentrating on sexual stimuli or by rejecting them. Muscle tension is also widespread, but much of this aspect of sexual experience can be controlled consciously as the individual literally works to reach peaks of sensation.

For convenience we divide discussion of the sex act into four phases: excitement, plateau, orgasm, and resolution.

Excitement

Initial sexual excitement can occur in response to any of a variety of stimuli. Sometimes a word, a gesture, a single caress, a picture, or even an odour is sufficient. In men, erection of the penis provides an obvious signal of excitement. The immediate cause of erection is relaxation of the muscular walls of arteries that supply blood spaces in erectile tissue of the penis. The large, thin-walled vessels that make up *erectile tissue* give it a spongy texture and permit it to enlarge.

As blood pours in from the enlarged arteries, the erectile tissue expands against a sheath of tough, inelastic connective tissue. Blood leaving the erectile tissue must pass into veins situated just inside the sheath. When blood is entering the erectile tissue fast enough to expand it against the sheath, these veins become compressed.

This compression, of course, obstructs the outflow of blood. With more blood entering than leaving, the erectile tissue becomes engorged and rigid, just as a balloon does when it is filled with water.

In women, increased blood flow to the sex organs usually occurs less dramatically. Often the first evidence of excitement is relaxation, enlargement, and moistening of the vagina. The vagina lengthens, partly due to elevation of the uterus. These changes create a welcome reception for the fully erect penis, even though insertion is possible when a woman isn't aroused.

Plateau

Numerous sensory nerve endings, particularly those within the bulblike glans, are stimulated as the penis is introduced into the vagina and rhythmically rubbed against the walls. Sensation and excitement vary during this *plateau phase*, which precedes orgasm. Engorged blood vessels in the outer part of the vagina may constrict the opening around the base of the penis.

Similar congestion of blood vessels enlarges both the *labia minora* and the *labia majora*, fleshy folds of skin that surround the vaginal opening. During this time both men and women experience a relaxation of surface blood vessels that produces a blush beginning at the base of the sternum and spreading upward over the face.

Erotic sensitivity is widespread in both sexes, extending to the breasts, buttocks, lips, anus, thighs, and often over the entire body. The *clitoris* of the female shares with the penis a common developmental history and basic structure. A mass of erectile tissue within the clitoris engorges and flattens and elevates the clitoris.

The role of the clitoris is difficult to explain. It serves as a center of sexual focus for women, and it is exquisitely sensitive to touch. Nevertheless, direct stimulation of the clitoris never occurs in any of the numerous positions of sexual intercourse. As sexual tensions increase, the clitoris withdraws under a clitoral hood. Although manual stimulation of the clitoris can help increase sexual tensions, it can be effective

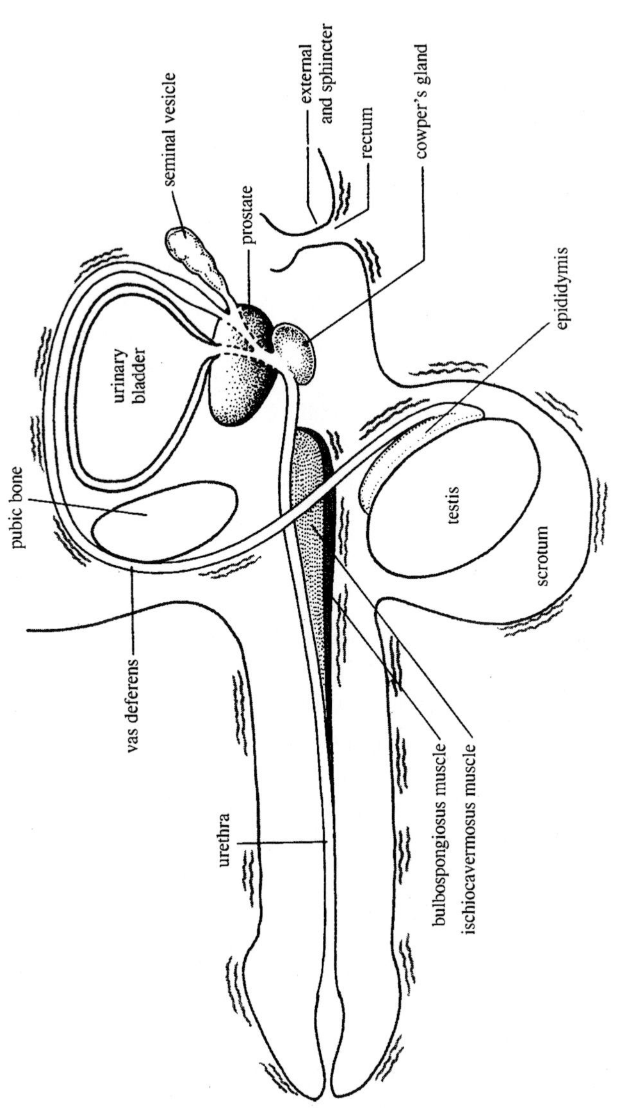

Figure 10.9 : Ejaculation.

through the hood, as well as when directed along the shaft of the clitoris.

There are as many fallacies associated with the size of the clitoris as with that of the penis. In neither is variation of size or position important. The vagina relaxes to accommodate any penis and can later close snugly against the shaft, no matter what its diameter.

Likewise, the sensual functions of the clitoris are the same regardless of its size. And since the clitoris is stimulated only indirectly during coitus, the slight variations in locations are inconsequential.

Climax

The sensations of *orgasm* (sexual climax) can be traced to rhythmic contractions of specific muscles. In the male, stimulation of the glans or of the tip of the urethra initiates a reflex. This reflex causes contractions in the walls of the vasa deferentia and the seminal vesicles, contractions that expel both sperm and glandular secretions.

Other motor nerve impulses produce spasms in skeletal muscles lying just outside the urethra between the prostate and the penis. The spasms massage the urethra and, when the sphincter around the urethra relaxes, help ejaculate the semen. Similar reflexes occur in women. The clitoris and urethra are the most sensitive to stimulation.

The skeletal muscles around the vaginal opening contract at orgasm. These muscles of the female are essentially the same as those of the male that massage the urethra and contribute to ejaculation. During orgasm the uterus and vaginal walls contract rhythmically 4-10 times at intervals of about 0.8 seconds. Probably such contractions aid the ascent of sperm toward the Fallopian tubes.

Whatever value the contractions have in furthering fertilisation, they are not essential. Pregnancy can occur whether or not the woman experiences orgasm.

Relaxation and Repetition

After orgasm, the muscle tension and increased blood in the various sexual organs gradually lessen. This is the period of *resolution*. Few males are capable of initiating another coital cycle immediately. Young men at the height of their sexual potency require about twenty minutes to recover. For others the time may be much longer. After an initial orgasm some women can immediately oscillate through several cycles of resolution and repeated orgasms.

Desire without Limit

The natural patterns of human sexual activity lie masked under many layers of cultural rules and expectations. Now that our society is more open to discussion of sexual habits, the pervasive nature of human sexuality has become evident.

No Respecter of Age

Studies have established that healthy humans often continue sexual relations well into old age. Many couples cease having coitus only when one partner suffers a severe illness. Perhaps the oft-heard tale that old age is sexless can be traced to the Victorian era. During that time the idea that no decent woman enjoyed sex may have led wives to terminate intimacies as early as possible.

But today menopause alters neither sex drive nor orgasmic ability in any predictable pattern. Reduced estrogen sometimes causes dryness and tenderness of the vagina and external female organs. Although the sexual appetite of males dwindles with age, many men are *potent* (able to maintain an erection) throughout life. Sperm production also continues. Men in their eighties have fathered children.

Health and Sexuality

Physical disabilities do not necessarily bar sexual activity. For example, there seems to be no more likelihood that sexual exertion will precipitate a heart attack than that any other aspect of ordinary life will do so. Those who survive coronary attacks are generally advised to resume an ordinary sex life when they return to other everyday activities.

Special problems face individuals with broken necks or spines. Because sensation involves centers in the brain, sex in the usual sense is impossible for these people. However, the spinal cord may remain alive, permitting men who are paralyzed by damage high in the cord to continue to respond to local stimulation of the penis.

They can ejaculate but without the usual sensations of orgasm. People with severe damage to the nervous system can offer the rest of us important insights into the real nature of love. Although handicapped in some ways, these people often establish deep intimacies and find a full measure of love and sexuality in physical contact even without coitus.

In fact, those whose daily activities are limited by severe physical handicaps may find their most important roles in love relationships. Such people often have more time and energy to expend on others than do those whose faculties are intact.

Nevertheless, it would be a grave mistake to suggest that most disabled people are incapable of an ordinary sex life. Injuries and disease that limit motion but leave sensation intact need have no important effect on coitus or orgasm. Families and friends should expect the newly handicapped to be as loving and sexual as ever. Sometimes sexual positions and techniques must be modified, but the emotions and sensations usually remain the same.

SEX WITHOUT REPRODUCTION

As everyone knows, sexual relations do not always result in pregnancy. Coitus is a means to reproduction, but that is not the only desirable outcome. Although some groups believe it unnatural and morally wrong to use sexual abilities in ways that preclude reproduction, the majority seem not to subscribe to this view.

Instead, they find the expression of love, the personal gratification, and the release from the tensions of life adequate justification for sexual activity. For this reason many people seek to uncouple sex and reproduction. And so they have done through the ages.

Contraception

Until recently the leaders of most nations considered large, growing populations in their best interests. (Unfortunately, some still do.) As a result, legal and religious pressures have been used to deter those who seek sex without reproduction. In the absence of *contraception* (techniques that oppose conception), people's sexual inclinations ensured population growth. Because of this pro-birth attitude, little effort has been directed toward learning how to manipulate human fertility. Consequently, the technology of contraception lags far behind what it might be.

Coitus Interruptus

Even without technology, thoughtful people have tried to control fertility. Perhaps the earliest and surely the most widespread practice is *coitus interruptus*. It was used in biblical times and is known almost everywhere today. Some people simply call this technique "being careful." It is probably the basis for the remark "If you can't be good, be careful."

As the name implies, coitus interruptus requires termination of the sexual union before it is complete. Withdrawal must occur before the man ejaculates. Use of this technique for birth control is based on the fact that there can be no fertilisation if no sperm enter the female tract. However, many men emit some sperm prior to orgasm. Furthermore, ejaculation onto body surfaces near the vaginal opening can permit semen to seep into the vagina. But because large concentrations of sperm are usually required for conception, the greatest risk is that the man will fail to withdraw in time.

Since coitus interruptus relies on attention and self-control, success depends in part on the man's motivation. Another problem is that sperm are left in the urethra after ejaculation, so reinsertion of the penis into the vagina carries a risk of pregnancy.

To avoid this risk, lovemaking is often interrupted, frequently before the woman reaches orgasm. Altogether, coitus interruptus is not the best contraceptive technique. Nevertheless, the failure rate is no higher than some for other contraceptive methods, and it has the advantage of always being available.

Condoms

Condoms are sheaths, usually of rubber. They are also known as "prophylactics," because they were long sold as preventives for venereal diseases in states where contraceptives were illegal. The condom is rolled onto the erect penis to catch the semen at ejaculation. Condom failure can occur from not leaving an air pocket at the tip; under these circumstances semen can easily leak out around the base of the penis. Or the condom can be lost in the vagina when the penis is withdrawn. Sheaths do rupture, though rarely. Used with care, the condom is an effective contraceptive device.

The Diaphragm

Until development of "the pill," diaphragms were the favourite contraceptive of welleducated Western women. A diaphragm consists of a rubber cap mounted on a circular spring. The spring holds the cap in place over the cervix. Used with a liberal amount of spermicidal (sperm-killing) jelly, a diaphragm prevents passage of sperm from the vagina into the uterus.

The fact that a diaphragm should be inserted no more than two hours before intercourse and left in place for six hours afterwards creates inconvenience. As with all contraceptive techniques, most diaphragm failures can be traced to human failure to use the method consistently rather than to flaws inherent in the technique. Since a diaphragm must be of the correct size, it must be fitted by a trained person.

Vaginal Chemical Preparations

There are a large variety of contraceptive foams, creams, jellies, and suppositories that contain sperm-killing chemicals. These spermacides should be used with a diaphragm, but they are better than nothing by themselves.

Rhythm

The rhythm method relies on the fact that a woman is fertile for only a day or so each month. Because ova usually remain viable for about a day and sperm for about three days, the period during each month when coitus can ordinarily result in conception lasts only four days on the average. Unfortunately, it is very difficult to determine when a woman will ovulate.

Generally ovulation occurs 14 days before the onset of menstruation. But just try to predict an event 14 days before another uncertain event. Addition of further days of abstinence to allow a margin for error reduces the safe days to precious few. Women can use their body temperature pattern to determine when ovulation has occurred.

Ovulation depresses the body temperature, but in the latter part of the cycle, temperature is elevated about 0.6°F over that prior to the ovulatory dip. Because of an inherent daily cycle in the body temperature and because physical activity increases heat production, the most reliable temperature measurements are those made on just waking. Nevertheless, worry, illness, and irregular hours introduce variability into the temperature pattern and can make its interpretation difficult.

Intrauterine Devices (IUDs)

Devices that are inserted into the uterine cavity are effective contraceptives. Unfortunately, as many as 30 percent of those fitted with an *intrauterine device* lose it from the uterus. Such loss is most common in those who have not borne children. To make matters worse, the woman is seldom aware the IUD is missing. Another disadvantage is that IUDs must be inserted by a physician or some other specially trained person.

Complications extend beyond loss of the IUD or pregnancy. Pelvic infections have been attributed to IUDs, especially during a pregnancy that occurs while such a device is in place. Severe bleeding is another problem. Furthermore, an IUD occasionally penetrates the uterine wall, and the repair is a major surgical undertaking.

Successful IUDs come in an amazing array of shapes. The mode of action remains uncertain. An IUD may act as a foreign body that stimulates uterine contractions, or it may attract phagocytic cells that attack sperm or the new embryo. IUDs wrapped with copper or infiltrated with progesterone may be more effective because of additional chemical action.

"The Pill" Oral contraceptives vary in their formulations, but they all contain synthetic compounds related to progesterone. These substances are synthesized from raw materials extracted from yams. Artificial progesterones suppress secretion of luteinizing hormone (LH) and prevent ovulation, just as does natural progesterone. Progesterones also alter the mucus of the cervix and of the uterine lining and thereby produce an environment inhospitable not only to sperm but to the implanting of embyros.

The standard contraceptive pills also contain estrogen, which inhibits the secretion of folliclestimulating hormone (FSH) and thus the development of follicles. In addition, estrogen suppresses the irregular bleeding that sometimes occurs when only progesterones are used. Usually the pills are taken daily for three weeks and then skipped for a week.

Withdrawal of the hormones permits bleeding, even as the natural decrease in hormones triggers menstruation. Some brands provide a pill for each day of the month; the pills for the fourth week contain only vitamins or some other harmless substance.

Not infrequently women experience side effects from oral contraceptives. Some side- effects are favourable; they include reduction in premenstrual tension, less menstrual discomfort and blood loss, and fewer skin problems. Negative side effects include weight gain, tender breasts, and headaches.

Blood clots occur with slightly increased frequency in women using oral contraceptives. Women over 30, especially those who smoke, have an increased risk of heart attacks if they take "the pill." Nevertheless, the danger of oral contraceptives is no greater than that of the childbirths that occur without effective contraception.

Other contraceptive methods, such as longlasting progesterone injections and progesterone-impregnated vaginal rings, have proved effective when tested. It seems likely that these and other new contraceptive techniques will become available not too far in the future.

Sterilisation

The contraceptive practices mentioned above are all temporary measures that usually have little effect on future fertility. But there is no assurance that surgical sterilisation can be reversed. This accounts for the hesitancy with which both physicians and patients approach sterilisation.

Vasectomy. Sterilisation is simpler in the male than in the female. Only a local anesthesia is needed, because the surgeon cuts the vasa deferentia just under the skin and ties or cauterizes (burns) the ends. After no more than a month, often much sooner, the man resumes normal sexual activities with no outward evidence of change. But now the sperm cannot traverse the vasa deferentia; instead, they are retained in the epididymides and are there phagocytized. Because most of the semen comes from the glands that join the vasa deferentia beyond the cuts, the ejaculate is normal in appearance. None of the nerves involved in sexual responses are harmed.

Complications of vasectomy are few. Occasionally a local inflammation occurs, apparently as the result of an allergic reaction to sperm that leak from the epididymis into tissue spaces. Because the sperm are not ordinarily in contact with the immune system, their components are not recognised as "self." It may be that vasectomised men risk rheumatoid arthritis or other autoimmune diseases.

If a vasectomy is performed carefully, there is a chance of reversibility. Some physicians have achieved 70 percent reversibility as measured by sperm counts. Nevertheless, most men with reversed operations father no additional children. Although they produce motile sperm, their semen doesn't function normally.

Tubal Ligation

In the female, general anesthesia and abdominal surgery are required to sever and tie the Fallopian tubes. The technique has been perfected to such an extent that only a tiny incision is necessary. Although the risk of injury or death from tubal ligation is slight, it is somewhat greater than from vasectomy.

Abortion

For a long time, abortion during the first three months involved scraping the uterine lining to remove the newly implanted embryo. Now withdrawal of an early embryo is achieved by suction through a tube. Neither procedure requires a general anesthesia, but there is always some risk of infection.

After three months of pregnancy, abortion may involve surgical removal of the *fetus* (well-formed young more than two months after conception). Alternatively, injection of a salt solution into the uterus will kill the fetus and placenta. Death of the placenta cuts off the hormone supply that maintains a normal pregnancy. In the absence of placental hormones, the uterine muscle contracts and expels the dead fetus and placenta.

All these procedures carry some risk to the mother, but if done properly in the first three months of pregnancy, abortion is less dangerous than childbirth. Abortions performed after the first three months are only slightly more dangerous.

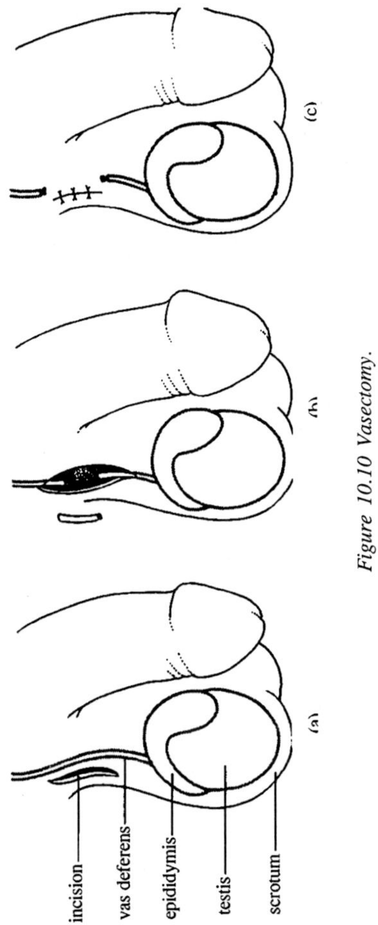

Figure 10.10 Vasectomy.

However, it isn't the inherent dangers of abortion that fuel pro-life campaigns. Opponents of abort ion argue that to abort is to take human life. For others the question relates not to the desirability of taking life at this stage but to its desirability compared with the alternatives.

The Private Practice

Traditional morality has limited sexual expression to intercourse with the marriage partner. Under the influence of this teaching, self-gratification through *masturbation* became abhorrent. In Victorian times, frightening disabilities were attributed to self-stimulation. One of the motives for establishment of athletic clubs was to provide an opportunity for exercise, so that young men could expend their energies in acceptable ways. Despite the concern about masturbation, there is no evidence that self-stimulation to orgasm is physically harmful. Although still vigorously condemned by some religious groups, masturbation is a common route to pleasure and to reduced sexual tensions.

The incidence of masturbation varies with age and such social factors as the availability of a sexual partner. Nevertheless, surveys suggest that at least 95 percent of the men in the United States and more than 50 percent of the women masturbate at some time. If they sustain injury, it is mainly from guilt.

Differences between Men and Women

Societies tend to prescribe specific social roles for each sex, but the nature of these roles varies so much among different societies that their biological basis is open to question. Although certain anatomical and functional differences between men and women are obvious, the biological components of other aspects, especially psychological ones, are unclear.

Development of Sexual Differences

Sexual differences are based on the distribution of chromosomes as will be detailed in other Chapter of this book. Briefly, each human female has two X chromosomes in every cell, and each male has one X chromosome and one Y chromosome. One of the two X chromosomes in each female cell condenses into a dense body. To establish the genetic sex of an individual, it is necessary only to examine cells and look for these bodies.

The sex of an individual is actually determined by the chromosomes received at conception, but body differences appear only gradually. The external form of the early embryo is neither male nor female. As shown in Figure elsewhere in this chapter, the external genitals of each sex arise from structures of an indifferent nature. In contrast, the early fetus possesses rudiments of the internal reproductive tracts of both males and females.

The genetic sex determines which of these embryonic tracts will mature. Thus adult males have vestiges of the female tract, and vice versa. Studies with laboratory animals indicate that secretions of the embryonic testis direct external structures into the male pattern, as well as supporting the growth of the male internal organs. In the absence of such secretions, the external genitals develop in the female pattern, and only female internal structures mature. Thus mammals develop as females unless a particular genetic makeup triggers growth and secretion of testicular cells.

The Basis of Sexual Behaviour

Just as the reproductive organs are initially neutral, so the embryonic brain is probably neither male nor female. Experiments with rats reveal that the presence of male hormone during a brief critical period a few days after birth patterns the brain for male sexual behaviour. This is true, regardless of the genetic sex of the animal.

Removal of either the testes or the ovaries from newborn rats followed by testosterone treatments for a few days results in adults that exhibit male behaviour. But if the ovaries or testes are removed at birth and no hormones are given before maturity, adults of either sex will show female behaviour in response to estrogen injections.

Thus development of female behaviour is independent of secretions from the embryonic gonads. Whether similar mechanisms operate in humans remains to be established. It is certain that the development of human sexual identity involves genetic, hormonal, and environmental factors. In people, learning plays a large role.

This fact is demonstrated by clinical studies of individuals whose reproductive structures are abnormal. The sexual identities of such individuals (as seen by themselves) correspond more often with the identities assigned by their parents than with their genetic or anatomical sex.

The role of learning in human sexual behaviour is emphasized by the effects of *castration* (removal of testes) in the male. Eunuchs who were castrated before puberty are incapable of performing the sex act. In contrast, mature men who were accidentally castrated after several years of sexual activity often remain potent for some time, even though their main source of testosterone is gone.

The Same Hormones in Both Sexes

This is a good time to point out that both males and females have hormones that are usually associated with the opposite sex. The adrenal cortex secretes testosterone as well as estrogen. When we speak of these as male and female hormones, we refer to the fact that males have more testosterone because of secretions from their testes.

Similarly, females have more estrogen because of contributions from their ovaries. However, the ovary also secretes some testosterone and the testis some estrogen.

It is tempting to try to attribute what we interpret as characteristics of one sex to the presence of hormones normally associated with that sex. In fact, adrenal tumors that secrete testosterone can "masculinize" a woman. The most obvious symptoms are increased facial hair and

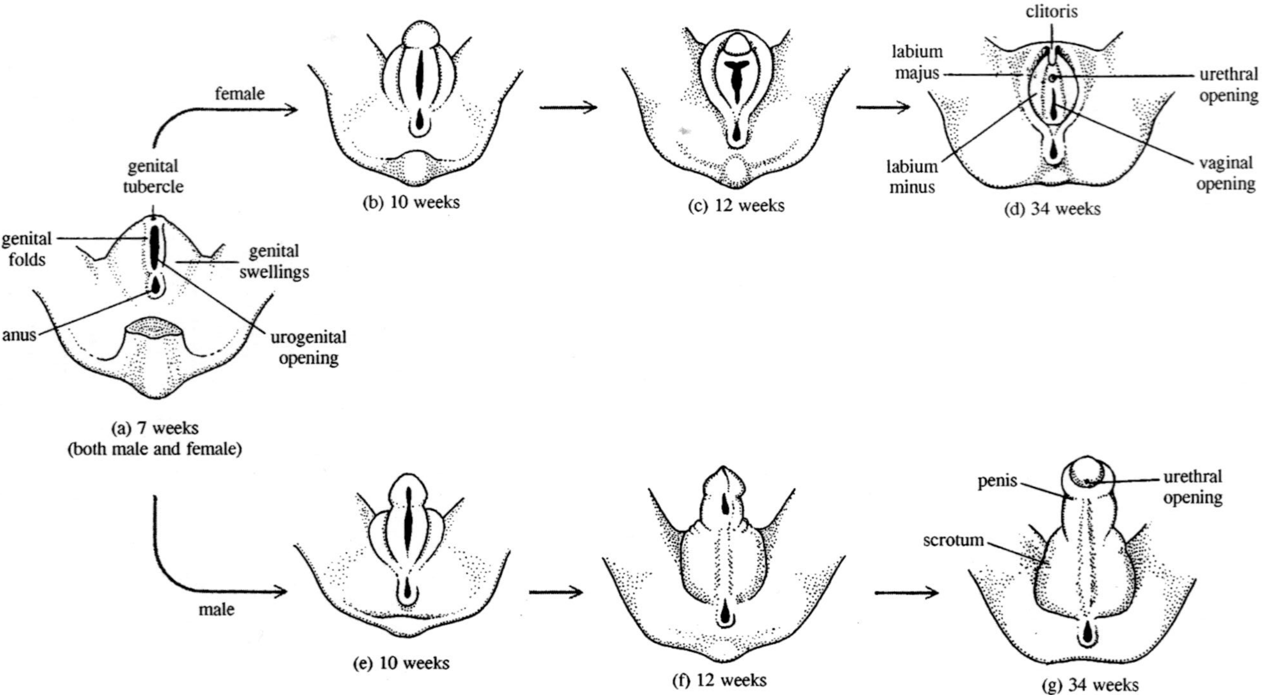

Figure 10.11 : Common Origin of the Male and Female External Organs.

depressed breast development. But in those rare individuals with atypical genitals, the adrenals are usually normal.

The hormonal similarities between the sexes extend to the pituitary. FSH and LH are secreted by the pituitary of the male, and they have functions in the male that are similar to those they have in the female. FSH stimulates development of the seminiferous tubules in the boy and maintains sperm formation in the man.

LH is necessary for the development and health of the interstitial cells that secrete testosterone. For this reason LH in the male is known as *interstitial-cell-stimulating hormone* or ICSH. Just as LH is necessary for ovulation in the female, it is necessary for release of sperm from the testis.

Sexual Preference

Attempts to offer a biological explanation for the variable attraction humans experience toward individuals of their own or of the opposite sex have met with little success. In present-day Western societies some individuals seem to be rigidly heterosexual, and a number are heterosexual in most of their contacts but occasionally exhibit *homosexual behaviour*.

A small percentage are almost exclusively homosexual. However, differences in sexual preference vary ever so slightly from one individual to another instead of falling into distinct classes. Studies reveal that a large proportion of adults in the United States have had sexual encounters with individuals of both sexes. In many other societies homosexuality is taboo or even unknown. However, in some it is widely tolerated or even prescribed under certain circumstances.

The innumerable variations in sexual preference suggest that many different factors may be involved. Although a genetic component has not been ruled out, there is no evidence that chromosomal abnormalities are involved in homosexuality. Furthermore, studies of hormone levels in homosexual and heterosexual individuals have shown no consistent differences.

Nonreproductive Effects of Sex Hormones

Aside from overt sexual behaviour, many psychological traits are often said to distinguish men and women. The biological basis of these traits remains an open question. Studies of sex-role learning demonstrate that parents have different behavioural expectations of boys and girls and therefore train them differently, both consciously and subconsciously.

Boys are permitted and even encouraged to be aggressive outside the family. Boys are also more often reprimanded with physical punishment. Perhaps this accounts for the fact that males commit most of the crimes of violence.

However, there is reason to accept the premise that some of the aggressiveness of males has a biological basis. Consider the behaviour of the males of other animal species. We recognise their aggressiveness when we use expressions such as "cocky" and "bully." On the other hand, attempts to correlate testosterone levels with social status or with aggressiveness are often unsuccessful. Socially dominant animals don't always have the highest testosterone levels.

But testosterone sometimes increases with sexual activity. Animals may develop higher testosterone levels when they become dominant and have more sexual opportunities. Sometimes it appears that the amount of testosterone may reflect behaviour rather than cause it.

Female hormones also have strong effects on the mind. Although testosterone injections increase libido (sex drive) in women, estrogen is important under ordinary circumstances. In most female mammals, *estrus* (heat or willingness to mate) correlates with estrogen peaks. For lack of satisfactory experimental evidence, we must base our understanding of the nonsexual effects of female hormones on observations of women during particular times in their lives.

It seems likely that the confident personalities of mature females may be promoted by estrogen. Perhaps this hormone serves women in much the same fashion that testerone does men. The influence of progesterone is more difficult to estimate. During pregnancy, when progesterone reaches its highest level, estrogen is also present in great abundance.

In females, marked alteration of sex hormone levels can have observable effects on the emotions. The severe drop in circulating estrogen and progesterone before menstruation appears responsible for the premenstrual tension that many women experience.

Some women also notice a restlessness when estrogen levels dip after ovulation. At childbirth, loss of the tremendous progesterone and estrogen production of the placenta renders many new mothers psychologically vulnerable. Unusual stress at this time can precipitate severe mental depression, particularly in individuals with a history of emotional problems.

It is quite likely that reduced hormones are responsible for the emotional upsets that sometimes accompany menopause. Of course, there are other factors involved. It is only reasonable to be depressed by the involuntary loss of reproductive capacity and to be reminded that youth is past. The headaches, fatigue, and insomnia that some women have may result from reduced estrogen. Ovarian secretion is irregular during menopause. At this time, fluctuation in estrogen is responsible for changes in the diameter of blood vessels near the surface of the body-the cause of "hot flashes."

Apparently the nervous system adjusts to permanently lowered hormone levels since the symptoms of menopause gradually disappear. In general, changes in hormone levels, rather than absolute levels, seem to have the greatest effect on the nervous system.

Hormones and Vigor

Lowered estrogen levels appear to be responsible for some of the characteristic aging processes in women. Effects are most evident in the connective tissues. For example, thinning of the skin is one regularly observed change. With neither sufficient estrogen nor testosterone, the bones become increasingly brittle.

The terminal tragedy for many women is a broken hip that never heals. Some physicians advocate replacement of the lost hormones through estrogen therapy; others fear meddling with natural hormone levels. Sex hormones are responsible for many average physical differences between normal men and women. The importance of these differences varies, depending on the situation.

Men are stronger than women, because testosterone causes muscle enlargement and makes muscle stronger per unit weight. This muscular strength combined with a larger skeleton and wider shoulders endows many men with a physique that can back up an aggressive personality.

In primitive societies this combination was surely valuable in protecting the family and in hunting game. Similarly, it is useful in the many presentday roles that require physical strength. On the other hand, a variety of traits, including larger adrenal glands and a circulatory system that can compensate rapidly for blood loss without risking shock, enable women to withstand physical damage much better than men do.

Even the extensive fat layers that underlie the skin and give the typical feminine curves to the body come in handy when a women is faced with cold or starvation.

When relieved from the dangers of numerous ill-attended childbirths, women tend to outlive men in our own culture as well as in many others. Apparently females benefit from excellent homeostatic mechanisms that evolved as adaptions to the rigors of bearing and suckling the young.

A GENERAL VIEW AGAIN

Although sexual reproduction is the rule for vertebrates and the predominant method among all plants and animals, what we have said about human reproduction can't be applied in detail to other species. Taken together, our reproductive adaptations are unique to our species. They evolved as they contributed to reproductive success.

In looking at other animals, we find that most are periodic in their breeding. In many vertebrates the testes shrink after the breeding season and develop again only as the next breeding season approaches. Ovaries may also undergo cyclic regression, especially in migratory birds in which a few grams of weight can be a burden.

Internal fertilisation is also the exception rather than the rule. In general, it is practiced by terrestrial animals whose young develop inside the mother or in shelled eggs. For example, in reptiles and birds the eggs must be fertilised inside the female before the shell is deposited. On the other hand, aquatic animals, such as fish, amphibians, and many invertebrates, practice *external fertilisation.*

Often a courtship ensures that the male and female are ready to discharge sex cells at the same time. Then the male simply sheds sperm near or over the freshly laid eggs. Much of the above also applies to plants, though in somewhat different ways. Like animals, plants have sexual reproduction and adaptive strategies that ensure that the sex cells come together.

Internal fertilisation has evolved in terrestrial plants as it has in terrestrial animals. You will find some of the details in other Chapter of this book. For now, remember that sexual reproduction is nearly universal.

11

DEVELOPMENT

Development adds a new dimension to the processes we have studied so far. While developing organisms are carrying on metabolism, maintaining homeostasis, and expressing the inherited patterns of their species, they are also changing from fertilised eggs into adults. To the usual life functions development adds organisation, growth, and the formation of different tissues from one cell.

The obvious complexity of these processes has attracted many scientists to developmental biology. We think you may share their enthusiasm and curiosity. The development of any organism is marvelous to behold. How is it that a fertilised egg can become a frog or a puppy or a human baby? Much of what occurs involves molecular processes yet to be understood.

But we do know that one of the first events is division of the fertilised egg into a mass of similar cells. This event is followed by a period of cell division, movement, and interaction that gives rise to distinct organs. Later divisions yield cells that become structurally and chemically specialised as they take on the characteristics of tissues, such as muscle, nerve, and bone.

After birth comes growth, maturation of reproductive structures, replacement of dying cells, and finally the degeneration of age. Although we are describing human development, similar processes occur across the animal kingdom.

FERTILISATION

Initiation of development begins with fertilisation of the egg by a sperm. Human sperm swim randomly, but contraction of the uterus propels the semen upward to the Fallopian tubes. The union of an egg with a particular sperm occurs by chance. But even though sperm approach an egg, fertilisation cannot occur immediately. First the sperm must penetrate the thick layer of follicle cells that surrounds the egg in the ovary and that stays with it after ovulation.

Enzymes from sperm acrosomesr digest the intercellular cement that holds follicle cells together. It is quite likely that many different sperm contribute enzymes that separate the follicle cells about one egg. If so, this may explain why the number of sperm ejaculated and their concentration in the semen are so important to normal fertility.

Although it may seem that production of any sperm at all should be sufficient to ensure fatherhood, many men are sterile if their semen contains fewer sperm than normal. A single ejaculate of a normal man may be a teaspoon of fluid containing about 400 million sperm. But infertility can be a problem if the ejaculate contains fewer than 50 million sperm per ml.

Male infertility may also be caused by sperm abnormalities. Once enzymes from sperm acrosomes have loosened the barrier of follicle cells around the human egg, a single sperm can fertilise the egg by entering the cytoplasm, flagellum and all. Soon the nucleus of the sperm and that of the egg fuse.

This union of the hereditary material from the mother with that of the father is but one aspect of fertilisation. Equally important, fertilisation results in *activation*, a series of changes within the egg cytoplasm. Our knowledge of this process in human eggs is scanty, so we rely on studies of other animals, such as sea urchins and frogs. In general, it has been found that a ripe egg is in a holding pattern, just waiting to be fertilised.

Once fertilisation occurs, the metabolic activity of the egg cytoplasm increases. Penetration by the sperm is also followed by cytoplasmic movements, especially in the surface layer of the egg. These movements mark the beginning of structural organisation of the new animal. It is important to note that the sperm contributes little cytoplasm to the *zygote* (fertilised egg).

And the genetic material of the new individual doesn't function immediately. Instead, fertilisation stimulates the egg cytoplasm to begin reorganisation. That this organisation is independent of fusion of the egg and sperm nuclei is evidenced by the fact that many physical and chemical stimuli can activate animal eggs in the absence of sperm.

For example, exposure to cold or to salt solutions may be sufficient to initiate development. Such development of an unfertilised egg is called *parthenogenesis*. It occurs naturally in some species, and it has been artificially induced in many others. Parthenogenesis is clear evidence that the sperm does not provide a pattern of development for the egg. Instead, fertilisation initiates a process determined by the egg itself.

DEVELOPMENT OF THE BABY

Beyond the zygote stage the new organism is an *embryo*. Cell divisions, cell movements, growth, and the appearance of organ systems all characterise embryonic development. In the human, fertilisation usually occurs within a Fallopian tube.

The zygote develops into an embryo as it passes along the tube into the uterus, where it embeds in the wall. By the time the embryo is two months old it has rudiments of all the usual organs and has thus become a *fetus*. During the remaining seven months, growth and differentiation produce the complete organs needed for independent function at birth.

Premature infants weighing at least 1 kg (2.2 lb) have adequate organs, so most survive. They need special care, including a uniformly warm environment, enriched in oxygen and free of disease microorganisms. Weight is used to predict survival, because length of *gestation* (time in the uterus) is difficult to establish.

If both mother and fetus are healthy, a fetal weight of one kilogram reflects about seven months of gestation. Babies weighing less than 2.5 kg (5.5 lb) are considered premature. Premature infants that survive suffer disproportionately from brain damage, mental retardation, nearsightedness, and other defects.

These conditions may result as much from the problems that caused premature birth as from the insult of meeting the world too soon. Frequently, prematurity is associated with multiple pregnancies or illness of the mother. Even more pregnancies abort spontaneously long before the fetus has reached a stage at which it can survive outside its mother. In these cases, embryonic defects are the most common cause of death.

Earliest Events

Immediately after fertilisation the new zygote undertakes a series of cell divisions known as *cleavage*. By this process the zygote becomes two cells, which become four cells, which become eight, etc. Although the nucleus is duplicated at each division, the cytoplasm doesn't increase in volume. The result is smaller and smaller cells.

At first thought, cleavage may seem so simple as to be trivial. The zygote is merely divided into a larger number of smaller cells. After

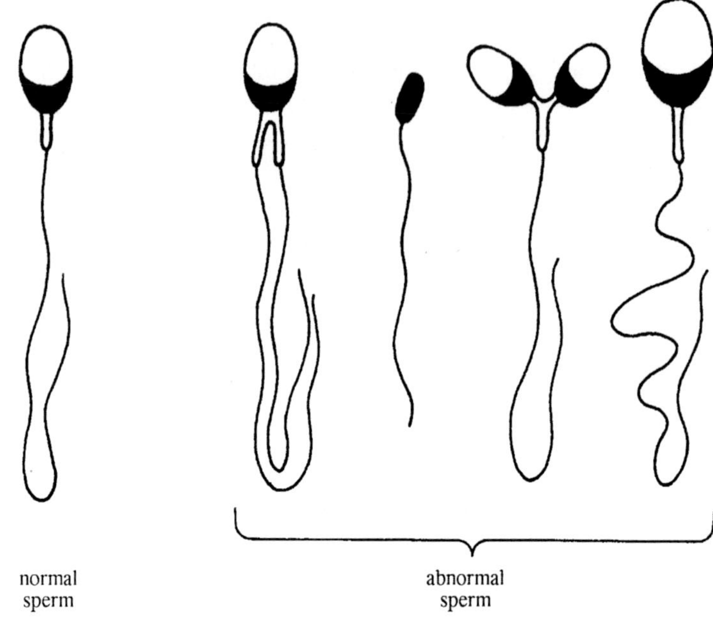

Figure 11.1 Sperm are not all normal.

all, the goal is a multicellular animal; numerous cell divisions are surely in order. This is true, but it is only part of the story. To understand cleavage we must further examine the egg.

The Egg Cytoplasm

Studies of eggs show their cytoplasm to be nonuniform. One point of nonuniformity is that the rate of cellular respiration is usually greater on one side of an egg than on the other. In many species cellular respiration decreases gradually across the egg.

As you might expect, mitochondria are most abundant in the region with the highest respiratory rate and least where the rate is lowest. Different parts of the egg cytoplasm vary in other ways. Often pigments are concentrated in one area.

Although the black melanin on the upper surface of a frog's egg may serve only to protect the cell from sunlight, we must recognise that if pigments are unevenly distributed, other substances that are displaced by pigment must be unevenly distributed, as well. Returning to cleavage, we note that these cell divisions cannot result in cells with identical cytoplasm.

If the cytoplasm of the zygote isn't uniform, the daughter cells must

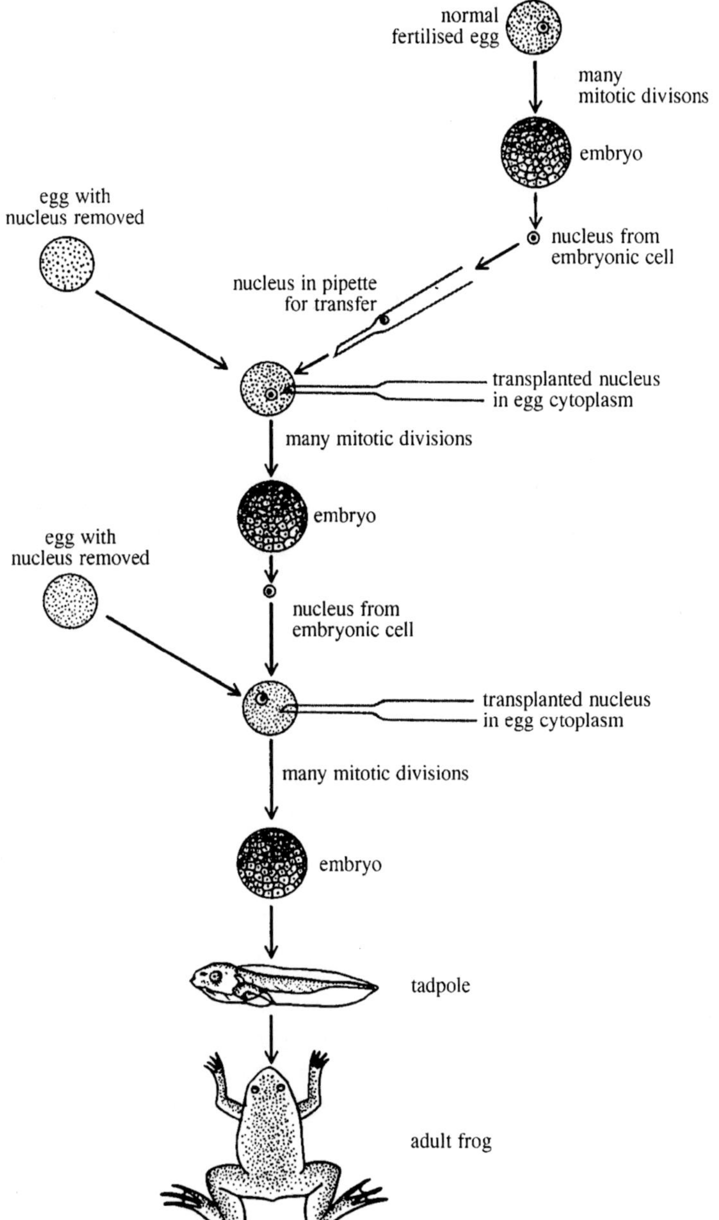

Figure 11.2 : Nuclear transplant demonstrates that mitotic divisions produce genetically identical nuclei.

receive different portions of specific substances when that cytoplasm is partitioned. Thus cleavage is the first step in the differentiation of cells.

The Significance of Mitosis

Cleavage divisions are the first of innumerable cell divisions during the life of an animal. These and most other cell divisions occur by **mitosis.** This process produces cells that are identical in their hereditary potential to the original cell. As you will remember, hereditary components of cells are carried in their nuclei.

Thus it is the *genetic* (hereditary) components of the new cells that are identical to each other and to the parent cell that divided. The fact that mitotic divisions create cells with nuclei genetically identical to each other and to that of the parent cell is of overwhelming importance. It means that all body cells have genetically identical nuclei.

This startling fact has been demonstrated beyond reasonable doubt. Indeed, each nucleus has all the genetic information necessary to form every structure and to perform every function in the entire animal. Here is the proof. When nuclei from cleavage and older stages of frog embryos are transplanted into enucleated frog eggs, the transplanted nuclei support development of healthy, mature frogs.

Even the nucleus from a lymphocyte can divide to provide nuclei for all the cells of an entire animal. So can the nucleus from a lining cell of the tadpole gut. Such gut cells are specialised for digestion and absorption; nevertheless, if a nucleus from one is transplanted into the cytoplasm of an egg, development may yield an adult frog.

These results are not a mere quirk of frog development. Similar conclusions have followed comparable experiments with insect embryos. There can be little doubt that even long series of mitotic divisions faithfully reproduce the genetic pattern present in the nucleus of the initial cell. Study Figure elsewhere in this chapter carefully, and be certain that you understand the significance of this experiment.

Returning to cleavage after having examined mitosis, we face an interesting possibility. If the nuclei are not altered by cleavage divisions, then the only differences created by cleavage must be in the cytoplasm. The most obvious aspect of this conclusion is that the far-from-uniform egg cytoplasm is divided again and again. As a result, some of the cells surely have quite different cytoplasm from that of other cells.

Gastrulation and Induction

Cleavage forms a hollow ball of cells, often called a *blastula*. The next step in development of most animals is *gastrulation*, so named

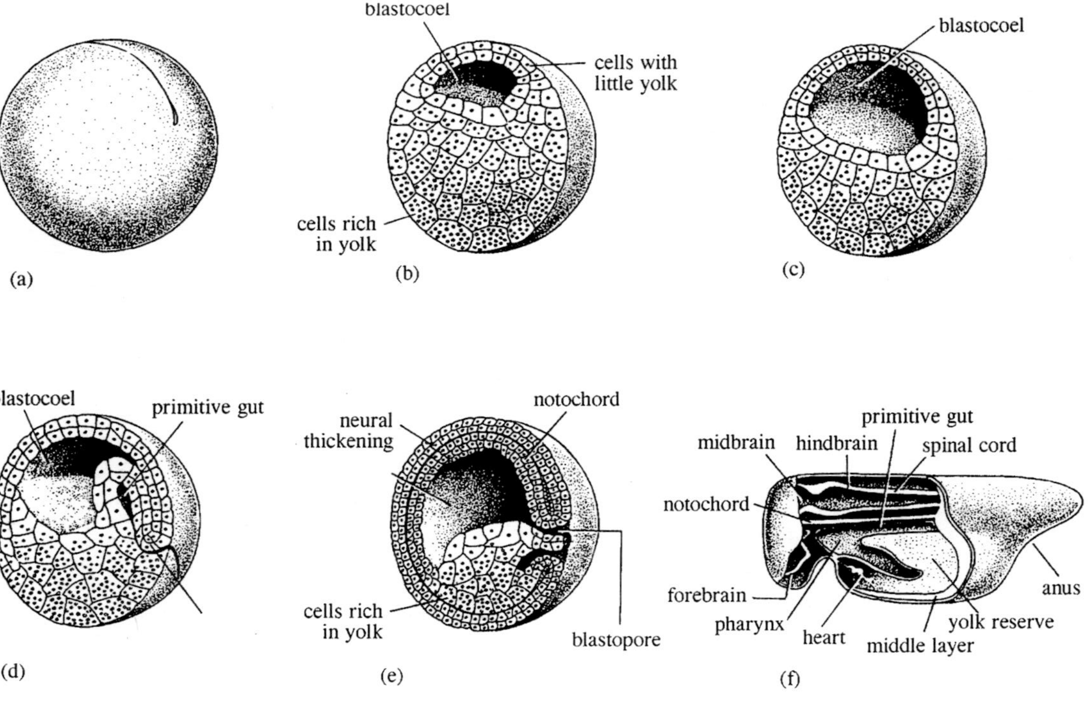

Figure 11.3 : Early development of frogs.

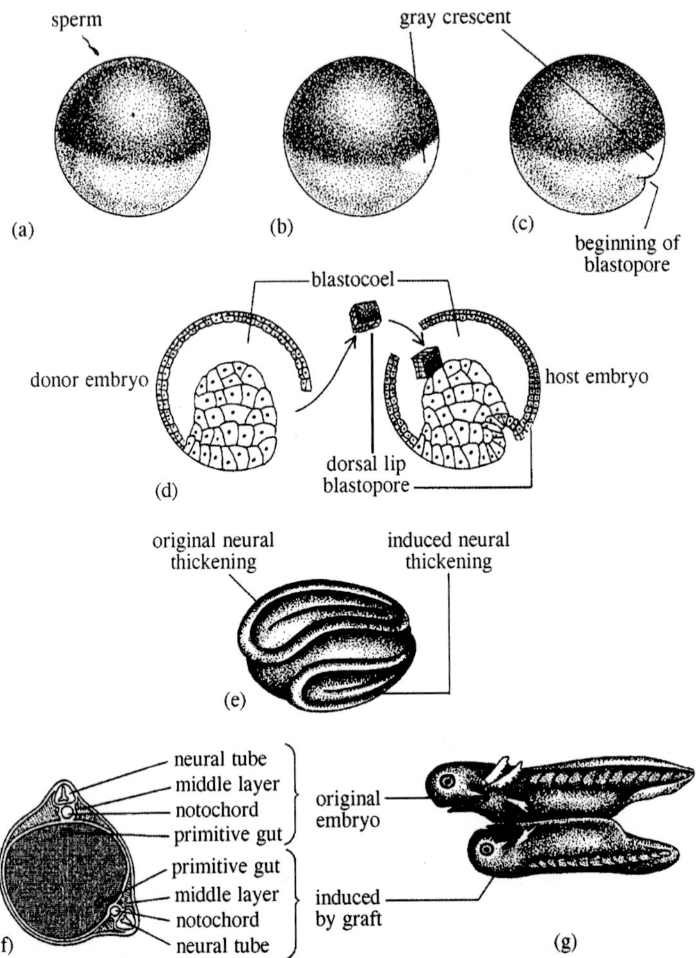

Figure 11.4 : Organisation of the embryo traces to a region of the egg cytoplasm.

because it produces a primitive digestive system. This process varies among different groups of animals, but in each it requires movement of cells and results in a multilayered embryo. The resulting layers each have different prospective fates; i.e., each will normally form specific tissues or organs.

Typical movements of cell sheets and the formation of new layers can be seen in frog gastrulation. Gastrulation involves movements of cell sheets or masses that alter drastically the relative positions of many embryonic cells. In contrast to the small differences between one cell and the next that are established by cleavage of the egg cytoplasm, gastrulation brings side by side many cells of quite different cytoplasmic properties.

Together with other facts, this relocation of cells provides a clue to control of development of specialised tissues. As we established earlier, the first steps of development are determined by the egg cytoplasm. We also showed that cleavage produces cells with identical nuclei but different cytoplasms.

All this makes sense if development is determined by processes initiated through the cytoplasm of various cell layers. There is evidence that this is what happens. Transplantation of particular regions of early salamander gastrulae reveals interactions between certain cell layers. Apparently one particular region initiates organisation of the nervous system and is, in turn, induced to form structures that give rise to the vertebrae, ribs, and associated organs.

Because one tissue induces another into special activity, interactions such as those illustrated in Figure elsewhere in this chapter are known as *induction*. Our understanding of induction is still limited, but the phenomenon is of great potential importance. If the cytoplasm of one cell can affect another cell, it may explain how cells with identical nuclei become as different as muscle, nerve, or liver.

Of course, such an explanation would imply that cytoplasm influences the nucleus. Although biologists have long talked of the nucleus as the control center, it seems obvious that the nucleus must respond to its environment. The cytoplasm surrounding the nucleus surely influences nuclear activity. The cytoplasm can in turn be modified by action of adjacent cells.

In the Uterus

Cleavage of a human zygote forms a berrylike structure. With further divisions, a space forms toward one side of the embryo, which is now known as a *blastocyst* (a modified blastula). The outer layer of the blastocyst is the *trophoblast*, and the remainder constitutes the *inner cell mass*.

Although the entire blastocyst results from conception, the embryo itself develops only from certain cells of the inner cell mass. It is within the inner cell mass that gastrulation and induction occur. The trophoblast contributes to the membranes that surround the developing baby during its long intrauterine life.

Implantation

By the time the embryo has become a blastocyst, it has reached the

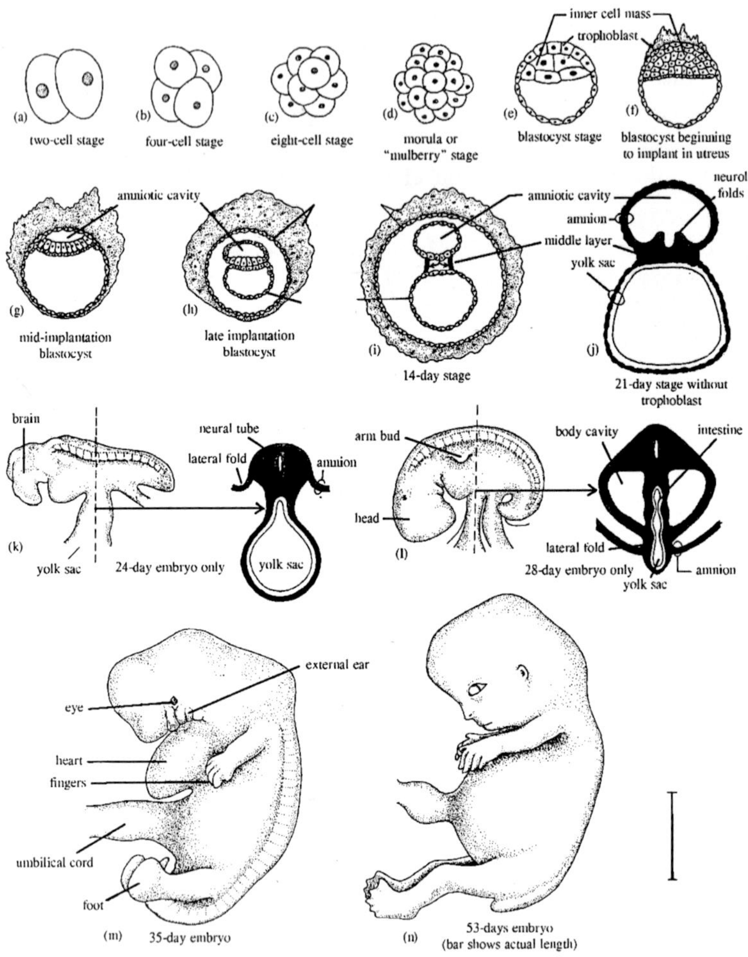

Figure 11.5 : Early human development.

uterus and is ready to attach there. About eight days have passed since fertilisation. During this time, the embryo has survived on nutrients stored in the egg cytoplasm and materials absorbed from secretions of glands that dot the lining of the Fallopian tubes and uterus. Now the embryo begins to *implant* in the wall of the uterus.

Implantation is initiated by trophoblast cells, which secrete enzymes that digest the uterine lining and prepare this material to be absorbed by the embryo. The maternal tissue responds to this invasion, but not in a defensive manner. Rather, the mother's cells grow and increase their content of glycogen, an animal starch that nourishes blastocyst cells. While the embryo is digesting its way into the uterine wall, the wall is also growing over the embryo. Soon the overgrowth of maternal cells and invasion of the trophoblast have buried the embryo deep within the uterine wall. This location necessitates rupture of the uterine lining before birth can occur.

Embryonic Organisation in the Human

During implantation fundamental changes are also occurring within the blastocyst. First a cavity forms in the inner cell mass. Because the upper layer of tissues will form the *amnion* (a membrane over the embryo), this space is known as the *amniotic cavity*. The cell layers between this space and the large blastocyst cavity become the embryo itself.

Of the prospective embryonic cells, those nearest the blastocyst cavity separate off and spread out along the sides to become the *yolk sac*. Eventually the yolk sac forms the lining of the digestive tract. Other cells lying in the midline of the embryonic region sink inward and migrate between the upper and lower layers.

These migrating cells eventually become the middle layer of the body, including muscles, connective tissue, and circulatory system. This series of separations and migrations constitute *gastrulation* in the human.

As the result of the gastrulation process, new layers of cells have arisen. Now the cells forming the floor of the amniotic cavity are induced by the underlying layer to rise in two longitudinal ridges. These ridges meet and fuse, forming a tube that runs the length of the embryo. This is the *neural tube*, from which both the brain and the spinal cord will develop.

Formation of other organs follows quickly. Soon the embryo takes on the appearance of a vertebrate. In this process the amniotic cavity expands and the lateral folds of the amnion move downward and curve under the embryo. This folding completes the three-dimensional form of the embryo and separates it from the membranes except at a narrow umbilical stalk.

The Placenta

The embryo in the early stages relies on substances it can absorb from the uterine lining, but it soon requires more effective nutrition, as well as efficient mechanisms for gas exchange and elimination of wastes. These needs are met by the *placenta*, an organ containing both embryonic and maternal tissues.

The trophoblast contributes to the fetal portion of the placenta.

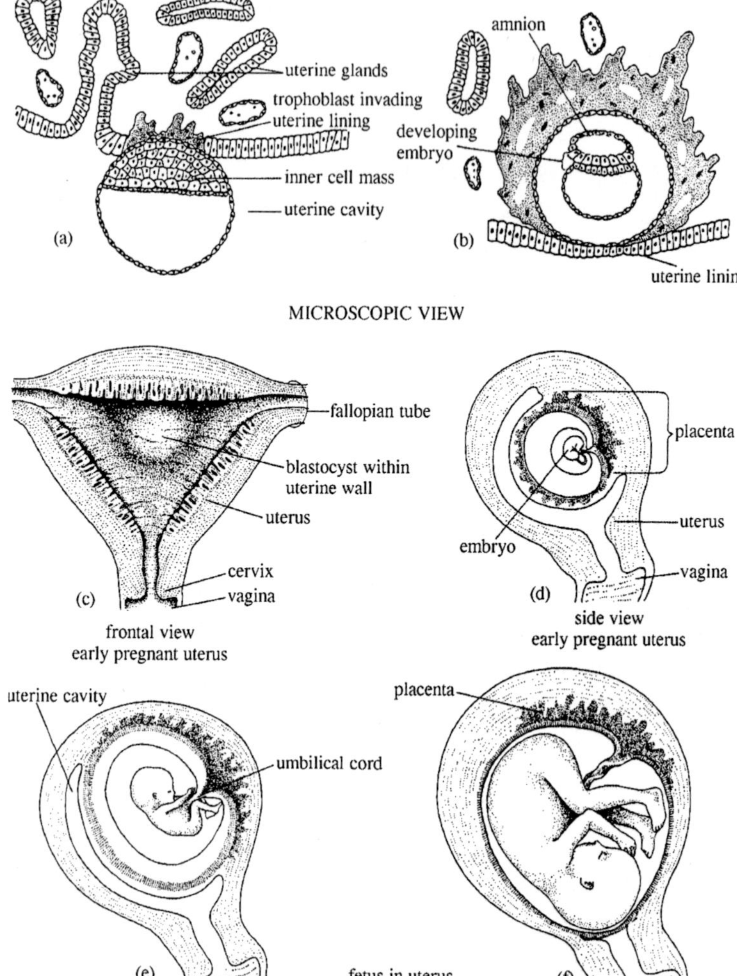

Figure 11.6 : Physical relationship between the embryo and its mother.

Blood vessels grow from the embryo into the trophoblast to form the umbilical arteries and veins. Soon blood circulates from the embryo, through the placenta, and back to the embryo.

Digestion of the uterine lining by the trophoblast and growth of the mother's tissue over the embryo eventually place the fetal blood vessels within pools of blood from the mother's circulatory system. Contrary to a popular misconception, the baby's blood and the mother's blood do not mingle.

Each has its own separate circulatory system. In the placenta the two circulations lie close together, separated only by delicate walls of tissue. Transfer of nutrients and oxygen into the embryo and removal of carbon dioxide and other wastes occur across a thin barrier.

Pregnancies Out of Place

Rarely, sperm reach and fertilise eggs that fall into the abdominal cavity. In a few instances in medical history this irregularity has led to the full development of a baby outside the female tract. Such development is possible because many tissues are capable of responding to the embryo and contributing to a placenta that will support a fetus.

Children that come to term in the abdominal cavity must be delivered surgically. If anything is to go wrong, the more likely possibility is that an embryo will settle down in the oviduct rather than migrate to the uterus.

These *tubal pregnancies* end abruptly and dangerously when the pressure of the expanding embryo causes muscles of the oviduct wall to contract and expel the embryo. The placental blood vessels are ruptured, and profuse bleeding results.

Motherhood

Childbearing is not a disease but a normal biological process. Nevertheless, medical supervision has become a pattern in the United States, and most babies are born in hospitals, often with the mother anesthetized. The desirability of anesthesia is contested by those who advocate "*natural childbirth*."

Proponents of natural childbirth offer classes that teach prospective parents what to expect and provide the mother-to-be with exercises that improve muscle tone and with drills in respiratory patterns that may aid her during delivery. It isn't clear whether the women who have such training have less pain for physical reasons or because of reduced anxiety.

But many parents trained in natural childbirth believe that it makes delivery a better experience, and that the less their child is exposed to anesthesia the better. A parallel social movement would return childbirth to the home and to the hands of the midwife.

Without doubt, the nurse-midwife can adequately attend to most deliveries. And there are advantages to home births, such as familiar surroundings and, sometimes, fewer infectious organisms. But a certain percentage of births inevitably require specialised medical personnel and equipment if the process is to be reasonably safe for both mother

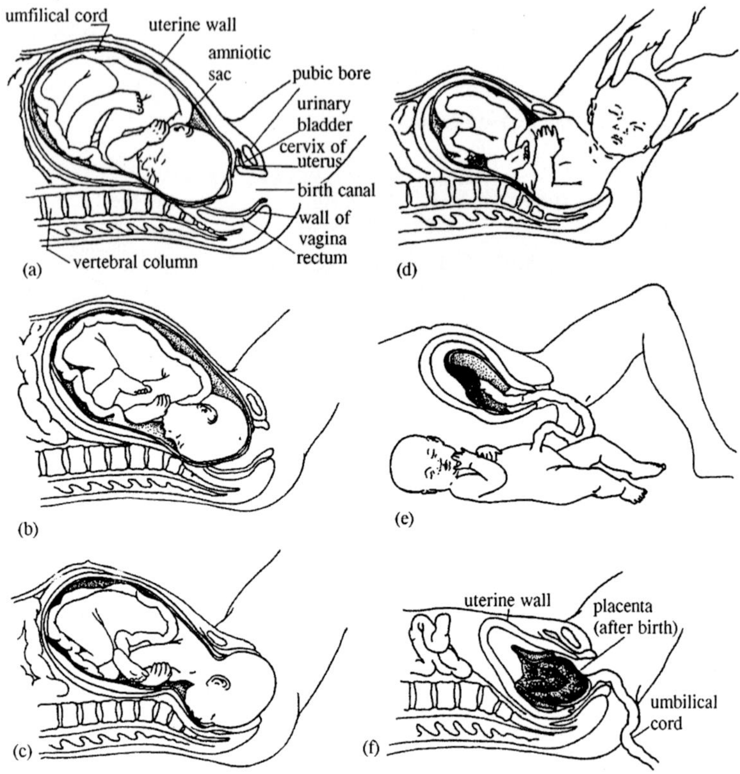

Figure 11.7 : The labor of birth labor.

and child. The trade-offs between often impersonal hospital experiences and old-fashioned home births can make the choice difficult. But in every case the prospective mother should have periodic medical examinations during pregnancy and be advised of the risk attending home delivery.

Normally birth comes after about 266 days of gestation. Four percent of births are late by three weeks or more, and more than seven percent yield babies classified as premature. Neither prematurity nor *spontaneous abortion* (loss of fetus) is likely to result from exercise, travel, or sexual intercourse during pregnancy.

In general, pregnant women are advised to continue an active life, to eat a balanced diet, and to get plenty of sleep. Avoidance of alcohol, cigarettes, caffeine-rich drinks, and other potentially harmful substances may be important.

Spontaneous abortion and low birth weight are especially common when the mother smokes during pregnancy. Similarly, even moderate alcohol consumption during pregnancy may increase the likelihood of physical or mental defects in the child. It is also wise for expectant mothers to use no drugs or medicines not specifically prescribed for use during pregnancy.

On Giving Birth

The birth process begins with a prolonged period of *labor pains*, caused by uterine contractions that usually force the head of the baby against the cervix of the uterus. After a while this pressure dilates the passageway through the cervix.

Dilation can take twelve hours, sometimes longer. During this time the amnion ruptures, and amniotic fluid is lost through the vagina. Eventually the baby is pushed out of the uterus by contractions of the uterine muscles, normally aided by voluntary contractions of muscles of the abdominal wall.

Further contractions of the uterine walls squeeze blood from the placenta into the baby before the umbilical cord is ready to cut. (The cord eventually shrivels up, leaving only a scar known as the navel.) A few minutes later, the uterus expels the placenta and the amnion as the *afterbirth*.

Because the embryo develops within the uterine wall, the uterine lining must be shed with the afterbirth. This accounts for the bleeding associated with childbirth. The exact stimulus for birth remains uncertain. We do know that the placenta produces large quantities of both estrogen and progesterone. Estrogen causes the smooth muscle cells of the uterus to enlarge and multiply.

It also increases the sensitivity of the muscle cells, causing them to contract in response to minor stimuli. Progesterone, on the other hand, inhibits uterine contractions. Indeed, this is one of its functions during pregnancy. Birth may be initiated, at least in part, by falling progesterone levels as the placenta ages late in pregnancy, *Oxytocin*, a hormone secreted by the posterior pituitary, also plays a role in birth. Physicians sometimes inject synthetic oxytocin to induce labor.

Birth Adjustments

The newborn must undertake for itself many functions that were previously performed by its mother. Whereas until now the baby has relied on its mother's lungs, now it must exchange gases directly with the air.

The baby must now also regulate its water balance and excrete wastes through its kidneys, instead of depending on exchange with the

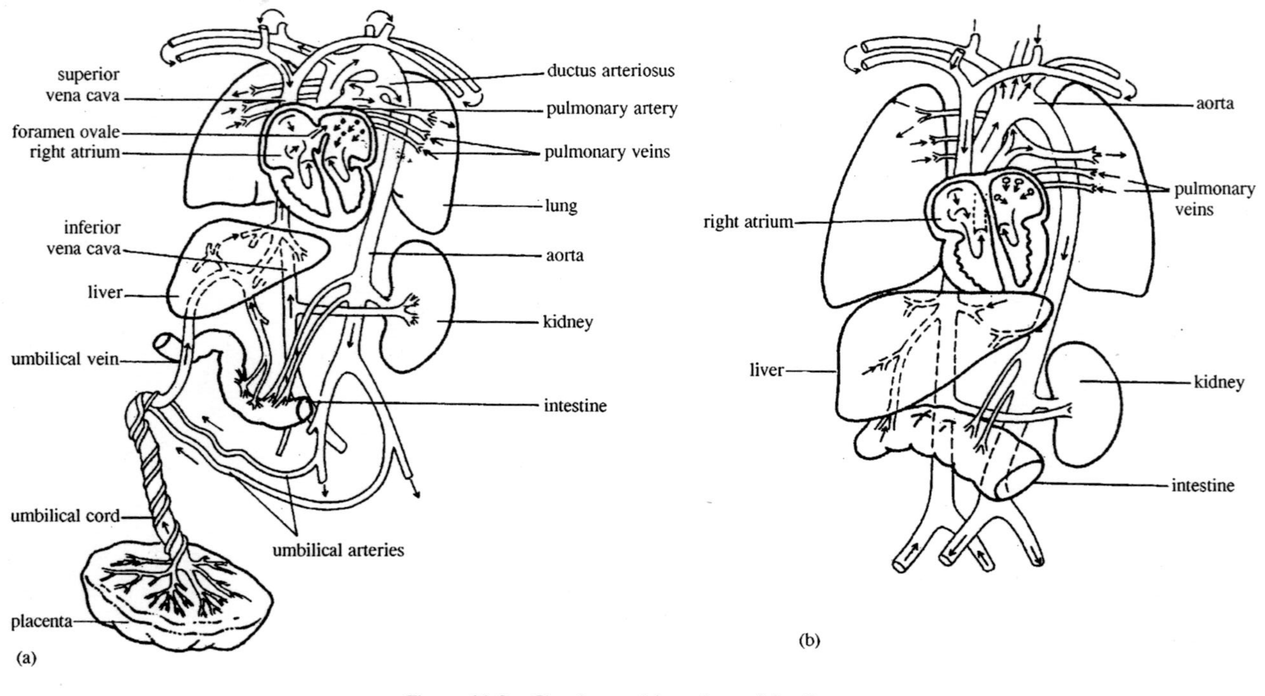

Figure 11.8 : Circulatory Adaptations of the Fetus.

mother's blood and regulation through her kidneys. And even though the mother provides the baby with food, it must now digest and absorb the food for itself.

Immediately after birth, the establishment of respiration has first priority. If the baby doesn't breath spontaneously in about 30 seconds, the attendant tries mild mechanical stimulation, such as flicking the soles of the baby's feet.

The gasp that usually results expands the delicate alveoli and transforms the lungs from solid masses into permanently frothy structures.

With the first breath, part of the fetal circulatory pattern becomes obsolete. During gestation, much of the fetal blood is shunted from the right side of the heart and the pulmonary aorta to the left side and the systemic aorta.

After all, the fetal lungs provide no gas exchange, so the flow through them needs to be sufficient only for development of the vessels themselves. With birth must come closure of these fetal circulatory bypasses. As soon as uterine contractions squeeze fetal blood from the placenta, the attendant ties and cuts the umbilical cord.

Then the baby is on its own. A change in the blood itself becomes evident a few days after birth, when most babies show *jaundice*, a yellow tinge to the sclera of the eyes and, in some cases, to the skin.

This unusual colouring is due to excess *bilirubin*, a pigment produced when hemoglobin is degraded. Abundance of bilirubin after birth results from a changeover in hemoglobin that accommodates the infant to new gas exchange conditions.

The fetus has a special hemoglobin that can draw oxygen away from the mother's hemoglobin. After birth the fetal red cells with this fetal hemoglobin are destroyed and replaced with red blood cells containing adult-type hemoglobin suitable for taking oxygen from air.

Temperature regulation poses another new challenge to the newborn. The tiny infant has a much larger surface for its volume than do larger humans. This large surface area promotes heat loss. So does the fact that many new babies lack insulating fat layers under the skin. To compensate, deposits of special *brown fat* can provide heat to an inadequately clothed baby.

Through an unusual metabolism, brown fat cells uncouple oxidation from ATP production' and release all available energy as heat. Taken together, the adjustments of birth place a tremendous strain on the newborn. Many defective fetuses survive to term only to die in the next few hours or days. Even healthy babies lose weight for a time, but after a short period they begin to grow again.

The Second Trimester: Organ Development

During the second trimester the details of organ structure begin to appear. Although the rudiments of most organs can be recognised at the start of the second trimester, during this time rapid tissue specialisation occurs. By the end of the second trimester the organs are distinctly formed. Most of those essential to life can function although they are far from the stage normally attained by the time of birth.

Fourth Month

During the fourth month hair begins to develop on the head and the eyebrows appear. The lips separate from the gums. The ears stand out from the head. The friction ridges which will later determine fingerprints become established. Minerals are laid down in developing bones so that these show clearly on x-ray films of the fetus within its mother's uterus. In addition to organ development, this is also a time of rapid growth. While the head remains large relative to the trunk and limbs, these begin to catch up. The fetus reaches about 14 cm (5.5 inches) in length.

Fifth month

Development of the nervous system is evident by presence of the grasping reflex. If the palm of the hand is stimulated, this reflex causes the fist to close. The fetus now exhibits other behaviour patterns. Many begin to suck their thumb about this time. Secretions of sebaceous glands of the skin and the shed skin cells combine to form a cheese-like coating that protects the delicate skin. Fine body hair helps hold the cheesy coating in place. By now the fetus is about 20 cm (7.8 inches) long.

Sixth month

During this period the eyelids start to open and the fingernails are well formed. By the end of the sixth month the fetus may be 25 cm (10 inches) long. Its organs are sufficiently developed so that it has a fairly good chance of survival outside of the mother if it is provided with skilled care. The use of a respirator after birth at this age is usually essential although the nervous system can control rhythmic breathing.

The Third Trimester: Tremendous Growth and Perfection of Organs

At the beginning of the third trimester, the fetus is skinny with red, wrinkled skin. At birth, three months later, the same baby will be much more plump. During the last three months it will have gained in weight from two pounds to about seven pounds. Thus its weight nearly triples during the last trimester. The weight gain slows the last two weeks before birth because the placenta begins to degenerate. A typical length at birth is 50 cm (20 inches).

Along with an astounding growth rate during the third trimester, specialisation of tissues continues so that organs are further developed. For example, the cerebral cortex takes on the convolutions and cell layering characteristic of humans. Brain waves can be recorded through the mother's abdominal wall be ginning with the seventh month. Yet development of the nervous system will not be fully complete until puberty, perhaps a dozen years later. Other organs of the newborn also differ in detail from the adult pattern but only the reproductive system is less developed than the nervous system.

By the time of birth the fine body hair characteristic of the fetus has usually been shed. Although bone formation has progressed rapidly, much of the skeleton is still cartilage. The bones of the skull do not yet meet in several places, often called "softspots." The sutures between most skull bones are still flexible. Thus the skull can be temporarily deformed to pass through the birth canal. In normal births this does the brain no harm and the skull resumes its usual shape within a few days.

Nursing the Baby

When a baby is born, the *mammary* (milk) *glands* of the mother's breasts must be prepared to feed it. The breasts of nonpregnant women consist mostly of fat deposits. The glands themselves are rudimentary. During pregnancy, estrogen and progesterone from the placenta stimulate growth of the glands.

Meanwhile, the same hormones suppress milk production by inhibiting secretion of *prolactin* by the anterior pituitary. Loss of placental hormones at birth removes this inhibition and permits production of prolactin. This, in turn, helps stimulate secretion of milk.

Control of Milk Production after Birth

Milk produced by cells within the breast accumulates in the glands and in their ducts. Nursing initiates a reflex that releases the milk. Nerve impulses pass from receptors in the skin of the breast to the hypothalamus. Here there are cells that have processes extending into the posterior pituitary, where they secrete *oxytocin*.

Once secreted into the blood of the posterior pituitary, oxytocin soon reaches the breasts. There it causes contraction of the glands, so milk is moved toward the nipples. *Adrenalin*, the hormone associated with the sympathetic "flight or fight" reaction, antagonizes the nursing-oxytocin reflex. Thus fright, anger, or other emotional upsets that cause adrenalin release also inhibit the flow of milk.

Antibodies in Milk

During the later part of pregnancy and for a few days after birth, the mammary glands secrete *colostrum*. This yellowish first milk is rich in protein, especially antibodies, and low in volume. Nursing immediately after birth protects the baby from infection through transfer of antibodies from the mother. True milk secretion begins on the fourth or fifth day after childbirth.

Importance of Neural Stimulus of Nursing

Continued stimulation of the breast is necessary for continued prolactin production. In the absence of nursing, the mother's milk supply soon dries up.

The neural stimulus of nursing also opposes release of luteinizing hormone (LH) and thus can prevent ovulation. Unfortunately this mechanism is not reliable enough to serve as a dependable birth control measure. In primitive societies, however, prolonged nursing may have some function as a birth-spacing mechanism.

Studies with the !Kung San reveal that births in this group are widely spaced without any obvious contraceptive mechanism. In that culture babies are constantly with their mothers, and they feed at the breast every few minutes. Some infants nurse almost continuously throughout the night. It may be this continuous stimulus of the breast that accounts for birth spacing.

Twins

Fraternal twins result from the fertilisation of two eggs by two sperm. Each fertilised egg forms a separate blastocyst, so each has its own placenta. Fraternal twins are no more alike than any other brothers or sisters, except that they are of the same age and therefore experience a more similar environment than do two children born at different times.

Because fraternal twins arise from two separate conceptions, one may be a boy and the other a girl, or both may be of the same sex.

Identical twins come from one fertilised egg that forms a single blastocyst. Either two inner cell masses develop, or less commonly-two embryos organise within a single inner cell mass.

In either case the developing embryos lie within one trophoblast and come to share a common placenta. It is possible, but not documented, that identical twins can also arise from separation of the cleaving

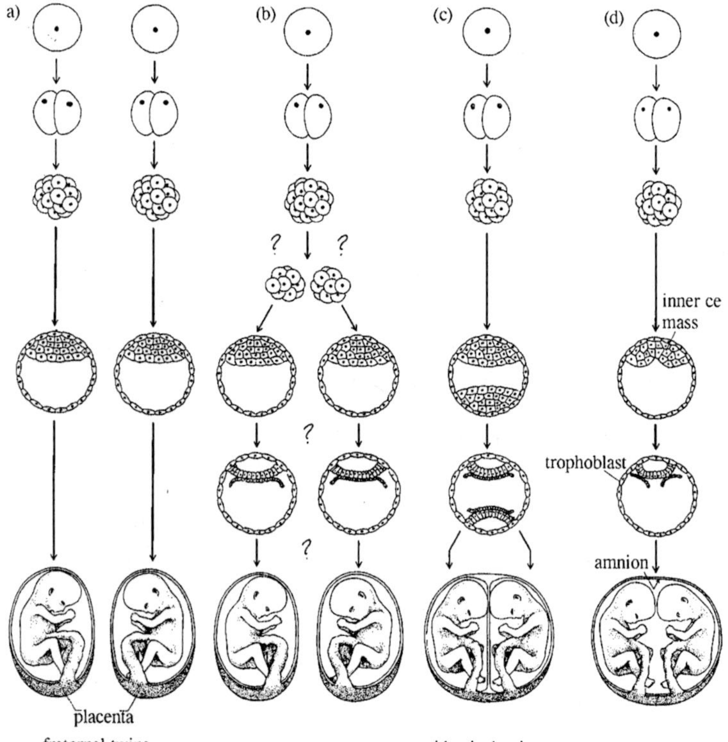

Figure 11.9 : How Twins Happen.

embryo into two parts before it forms a blastocyst. Such identical twins would have separate placentas. Except for births under this possible but unsubstantiated condition, the physician or midwife attending births can determine whether twins are identical or fraternal merely by noting whether the afterbirth consists of one placenta or two.

Multiple births are not randomly distributed. The frequency of fraternal twins varies among races; the incidence is higher among Caucasians than among the Japanese. Studies of families also suggests that the tendency for women to ovulate two eggs the same month and thus to have fraternal twins seems to be inherited.

Births of identical twins are more common in older mothers. Recently treatments for female sterility that is caused by a sluggish pituitary have led to numerous cases of three or more simultaneous births. This results from the fact that the drugs sometimes cause the ovulation of several eggs at once.

Birth Defects

The dread of malformed bodies is so great that almost all societies have pregnancy taboos designed to protect the unborn child. But despite magic and medicine, a large portion of conceptions produce defective embryos. Estimates range from 10 to 80 percent. These figures include both pregnancies that terminate in spontaneous abortions and those that deliver babies with minor to severe handicaps.

The large range in the estimates reflects disagreement on the frequency and cause of very early spontaneous abortions. It is established that many embryos abort so early that the mother doesn't realise she has been pregnant. But how often this happens we are unsure.

Although genetic defects are a major cause of abnormal embryonic development, nutritional deficiencies, infections, drugs, and maternal disease also contribute to the problem.

Table 11.1 : Congenital Defects in Humans.

Time of Recognition	*% of Total Conceptions*
Causing spontaneous abortions	5
Stillborn	0.5
Recognised at live birth	1.5
Detected later	3
Total Incidence	10%

Viruses

Rubella (German measles), influenza, smallpox, and other viruses can penetrate the placenta and infect the fetus while it is in the uterus. Often the fetus dies as the result of infection, and the pregnancy comes to an early end. But in many cases only specific embryonic tissues die.

For instance, rubella can damage cells that form the sense organ of the inner ear or those that should form the lens of the eye. As a result the child is deaf, or its vision is clouded by cataracts. Congenital malformations of the heart also appear in as many as 80 percent of those that survive *prenatal* (before birth) *rubella*.

As a reflection of crucial steps in development, viral diseases are most serious at certain stages. For rubella, the most dangerous time is between the fourth and the twelfth week of pregnancy.

Susceptibility

Studies of palate development in two inbred strains of mice demons-

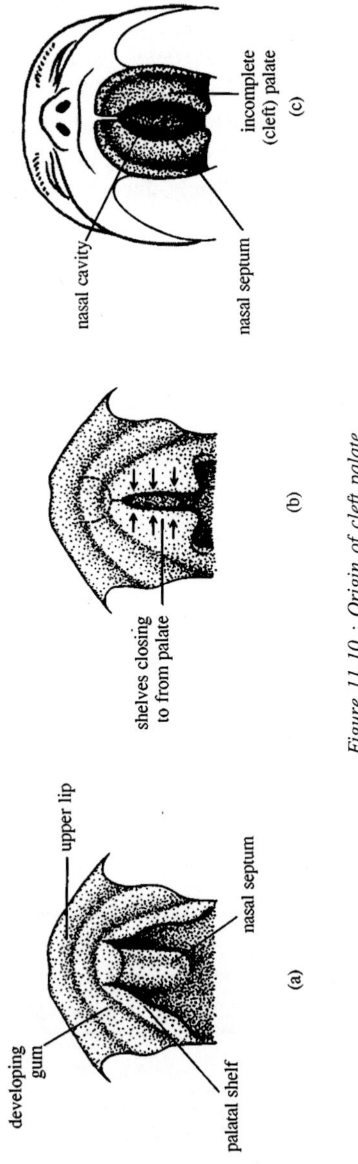

Figure 11.10 : Origin of cleft palate.

trate the interaction of genetic and environmental influences on birth defects. Large doses of the adrenal hormone *cortisone*, given at specific times, results in *cleft palate* in 100 percent of the offspring of one mouse strain known as A/J. The same doses given to C57BL mice at the same stage of pregnancy have no effect.

As shown in Figure elsewhere in this chapter, cleft palate results from failure of the two palatal shelves to fuse together. Formation of a continuous palate is possible only during a certain stage. After that time, growth of the head carries the palatal shelves apart faster than they can grow toward each other. The growth of palatal shelves in A/J mice is always slower than in C57BL mice.

Consequently, palatal fusion occurs later in the A/J strain. There is a high incidence of cleft palate in the A/J strain, even under the best

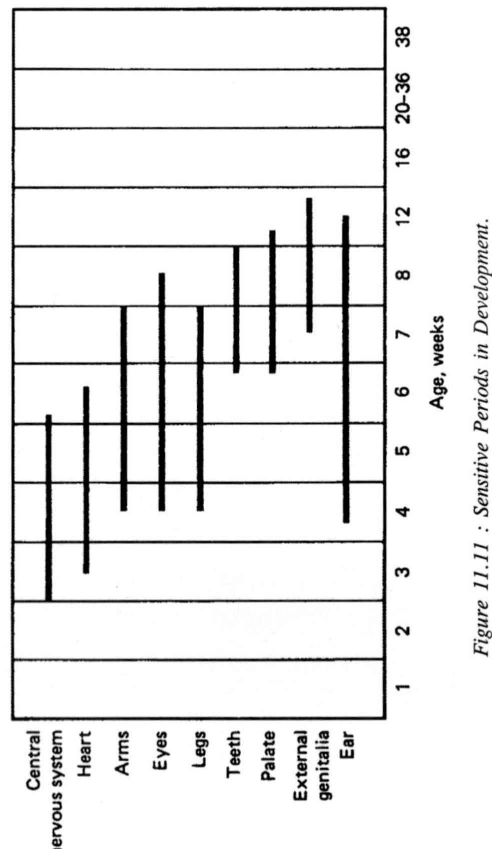

Figure 11.11 : Sensitive Periods in Development.

conditions. When administration of cortisone slows palatal growth further, the shelves never fuse. In contrast, the palatal shelves of C57BL mice grow fast.

In this strain, fusion occurs even in the presence of experimental doses of cortisone. Thus a physiological factor, cortisone, causes a birth defect in one strain but not in another. The inherited growth characteristics of A/J mice make them particularly susceptible to cortisone.

Sensitive Periods

Obviously cortisone can act on A/J mouse embryos only after certain developmental stages are reached and before the shelves have fused. Therefore A/J mouse embryos are sensitive to cortisone only during a particular period. Such sensitive periods are characteristic of embryonic development. Because these periods reflect major organisational events, they are confined to early development.

The embryonic stages of human development most susceptible to deformity occur between two and six weeks of gestation. It is during this period that most major malformations originate. The births of flipper-limbed babies to women who used the sedative thalidomide illustrate this problem.

It is tragic that the embryo reaches its most sensitive stages before the mother may be aware that she is pregnant. Thus the precautions expectant mothers take come too late to protect the baby from most environmental harm. The only answer to this problem is for women who may conceive to always take the same precautions that they would if they knew they were pregnant.

Environmental factors are not the only ones that increase the likelihood of bearing a defective child. As we will discuss in the following chapter, women in their late thirties or older often produce eggs with chromosomal defects.

The presence of certain inherited disease on either or both sides of the family also increases the risk of a defective baby. Thus some prospective parents are especially concerned about the fetus. Many choose to use *amniocentesis* to determine whether their baby will be normal.

Amniocentesis can reveal genetic defects present in all the cells of the fetus but not malformations that have been induced by the action of environmental factors at a particular stage of development. Since 96 percent of the fetuses checked by amniocentesis prove genetically normal, this procedure relieves a great deal of anxiety.

It also can prevent the choice of abortion in high-risk cases, for

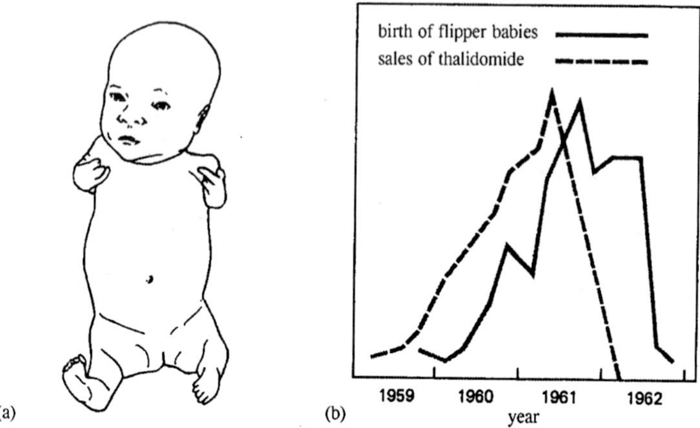

Figure 11.12 : Sensitivity of human embryos to thalidomide.

more often than not the fetus proves healthy. The procedure of amniocentesis itself is usually harmless, but its use increases slightly the chance of a spontaneous abortion. Reports that fetal cells regularly enter the mother's blood have led to suggestions for simpler methods to isolate fetal cells for laboratory study. Someday it may be necessary only to draw blood from the mother's arm.

DEVELOPMENT AS A LIFELONG PROCESS

Development doesn't stop at birth. Characteristic changes occur throughout our lifespan. At least some of these changes reflect selection of traits that favour continuation of the species and are clearly inherited by us all.

Growth

A graph of the weight of an animal plotted against its age may yield an S-shaped curve. The slow increase at the beginning reflects initial organisation of the embryo and adjustment to the environment. Once the basic structures are established, the embryo grows at an increasing rate until a maximum rate is reached.

After a time, the growth rate begins to decrease, and eventually growth comes to an end. Of course, many animals deviate from this theoretical growth curve. For example, accumulation of fat and its loss during famine can distort the curve. So does the tendancy for older organisms to contain less water per cell than younger animals do. In fact, growth curves are most meaningful if they reflect the number of cells in the organism.

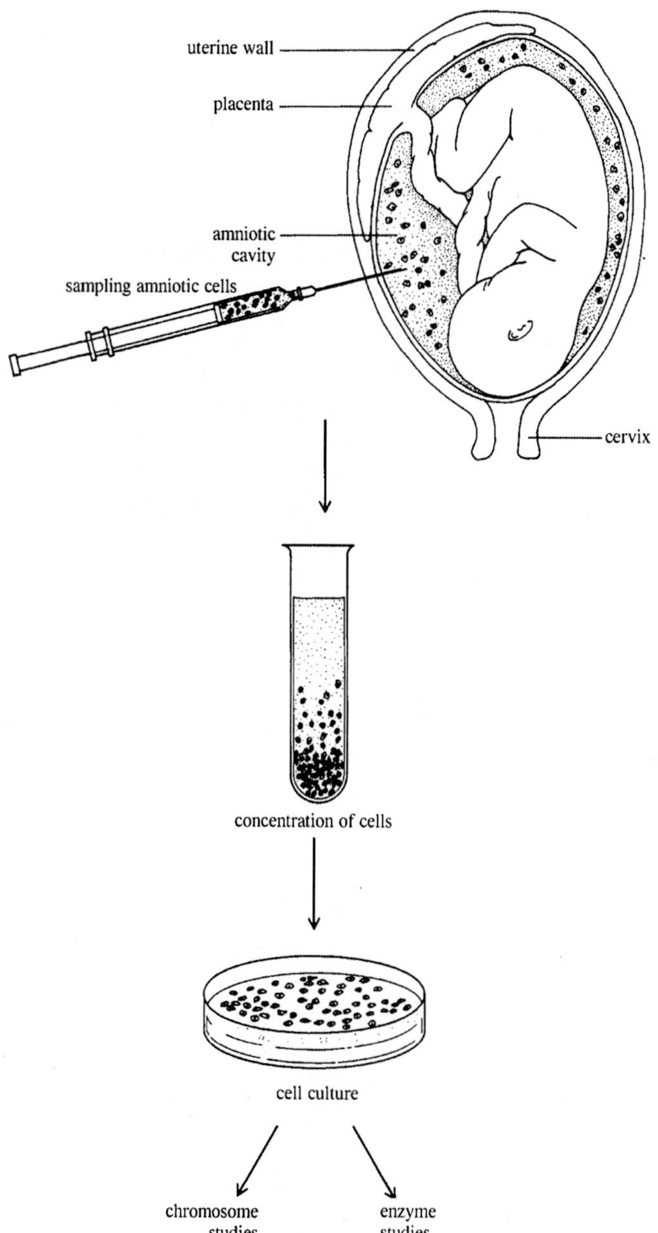

Figure 11.13 : Amniocentesis—Checking out the unborn.

However, since it is impractical to count the cells in an animal, growth curves are often based on weight, length, or height. For people, growth curves based on height vary from the general S-shaped curve in two ways. First, the newborn has already undergone the initial adjustments and entered a stage of rapid growth.

This growth tapers off before birth but is later resumed. Secondly, the human growth curve shows a small hump known as the *adolescent growth spurt*. It appears at about the time the secondary sexual characteristics develop.

In males the increase in height is accompanied by lengthening of the penis, enlargement of the testes, and appearance of the characteristic male pattern of pubic hair. Breast development occurs during the adolescent growth spurt of females. Menstruation begins near the end of the spurt.

Of course, different parts of the body grow at different rates. The brain gets its growth early, as shown by the fact that children have large heads in proportion to their bodies. Probably you have noted that cartoonists use this differences to distinguish the figures of children from those of adults.

The early, rapid growth of the nervous system is necessary, because that system must be nearly complete before the child begins important learning tasks. In contrast, the reproductive system grows very slowly until just before sexual maturity.

In the sense that cell division continues, growth occurs throughout life. Although nerve and skeletal muscle cells cannot divide, perhaps because they are too specialised, most other tissues can replace old cells with new ones. In some tissues, such as the epithelium of the skin, division is confined to particular cells.

In many organs growth is limited to connective tissue that forms scars. This is true in the heart. In yet other organs, most or all cells can divide. This is so for the liver, in that removal of a portion may be followed by appearance of new, properly organised lobes.

In considering growth, we must point out that addition of new cells is only one aspect of development. The new cells are useful only when they have *differentiated* (specialised) into characteristic tissues that function in cooperation with others in the body. Control of this process of differentiation is one of the intriguing problems facing biologists today.

Aging

Some biologists view aging as a part of development. In other words, aging may be programmed into the individual just as are other phases of development. There is good evidence that aging has some inherited basis. For example, the life spans of identical twins coincide more closely than do those of fraternal twins of the same sex.

The life spans of children correlate well with those of their parents. Furthermore, there is an inherited disease, *progeria*, in which aging occurs prematurely. Individuals with progeria suffer degenerative changes, such as atherosclerosis, so early that death often comes in childhood.

To the degree that aging is genetically controlled, there may be little we can do to prevent its onset. The changes involved are too widespread to result from a single metabolic defect that could be cured as diabetes is "cured" by the regular injection of insulin.

According to another view, the degeneration of aging results from some random action, as by radiation or other universally present environmental factors. Perhaps defects accumulate because of accidents during mitosis. But whatever the role of the environment in aging, it seems likely that our life style may hurry or retard degeneration. Diet, smoking, alcohol abuse, emotional stress, and physical exertion may all have a role.

While biologists ponder the basic causes of aging, a desire for eternal youth lies deep within us. It supports a flourishing trade in popular literature that offers to tell us how to retain or regain youth. Some people submit to extreme procedures in the hope of being young again. During the 1930s transplantation of monkey testes into old men was a fad. More recently people have sought restored youth through injections of cells from young animals, such as lambs.

Such farfetched schemes thrive because medical science has nothing to offer. Although control of infectious disease has increased the average human life span dramatically in this century, the maximum life span remains unchanged. People are becoming more aware of the infirmities of age as an ever-larger proportion of the population survive long enough to be affected.

Death

The more we learn about ourselves and other organisms, the harder it is to come up with an absolute definition of either life or death. A case in point concerns human cells that outlive the individual. Just like bacteria or yeast, many kinds of human cells can be grown in bottles and flasks if supplied with proper nutrients.

The best known human cell line was derived from the cervical cancer of a Baltimore woman who died many years ago. Biologists call

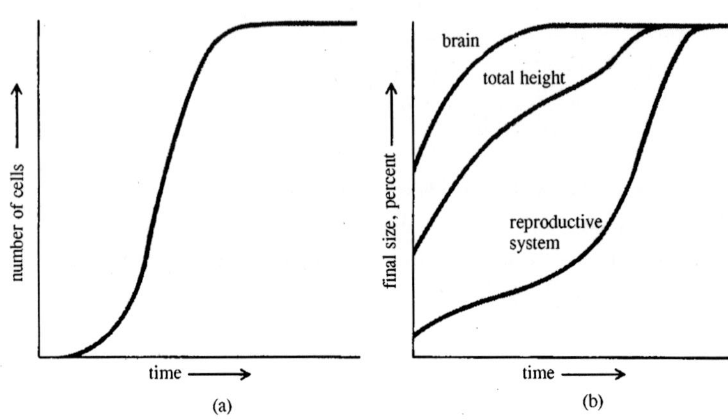

Figure 11.14 : Growth curves.

these *HeLa cells* because, according to tradition, the woman's name was Henrietta Lacks.

HeLa cells are extemely easy to culture. If even a very small number of them contaminate other cultures, the HeLa cells may overgrow the rightful inhabitants of the container. Still, no one would deny that Henrietta Lacks is dead just because her cells multiply in laboratories around the world.

The Essence

Most people would agree that the essence of life in humans or other animals is centered in the brain and in the mind. But even severe brain damage may have little impact on such "vital" signs as breathing and heartbeat.

And although the effort is often futile and wasteful, a heart-lung machine can support the body for some time after most of the brain has ceased to work. No matter how many functions of the body are replaced with mechanical devices or transplants, no substitute nervous system can recreate a mind.

If a brain could be transplanted, the identify of the individual would very likely pass with the brain. For this reason, absence of electrical activity in the brain for some critical period may be the best criterion of death.

The End

Even though the brain, heart, and lungs no longer function, all the body cells do not die instantly. Just as it is possible to take a pint of blood from a healthy person and refrigerate it for weeks before using it in a transfusion, so it is possible to take healthy tissues, such as the cornea of the eye, from the body of someone who has recently died and use them as grafts in living people.

Once the person is dead, the body cools slowly. How slowly depends on weight, clothing, and the environment. Under ordinary conditions, about 24 hours pass before the body reaches room temperature. Within a few hours of death, blood begins to accumulate by gravity on the lower side of the body.

Because deoxygenated hemoglobin is bluish-red, the lower surfaces take on a purplish hue. As individual body cells die, their lysosomes disintegrate and release enzymes that destroy other cell components. Once the epithelial cells fall apart and phagocytes cease their work, the microorganisms of the normal flora invade unchecked.

As our developmental cycle comes full turn, the chemical elements that compose our bodies move on in the biogeochemical cycles" that make us one with the biosphere.

DEVELOPMENT: CHALLENGE OF TODAY

How a single cell becomes a human being is a puzzle that is far from solved. Much of what we know is in the "embryonic" stage. Our knowledge is mostly descriptive.

We can observe the sequence of changes, but how it happens eludes us. In this chapter, we spoke of induction and of the interactions of cytoplasm and nucleus, but there are no clear explanations. We aren't even certain what triggers cells to divide.

More perplexing is the question of how cells become as different as neurons and bone cells. The answer surely involves molecules and heredity, but exact pathways remain unknown. Although we offer no details on developmental mechanisms, we can share with you a general background in how inheritance is determined and expressed.

With such information you should be able to follow the story of developmental biology as it unfolds in the years ahead. For this introduction to heredity, turn to the following chapters.

INDEX

B

C

D

E

J

K

L

M

N

O

P

R

S

T

U

V